Release

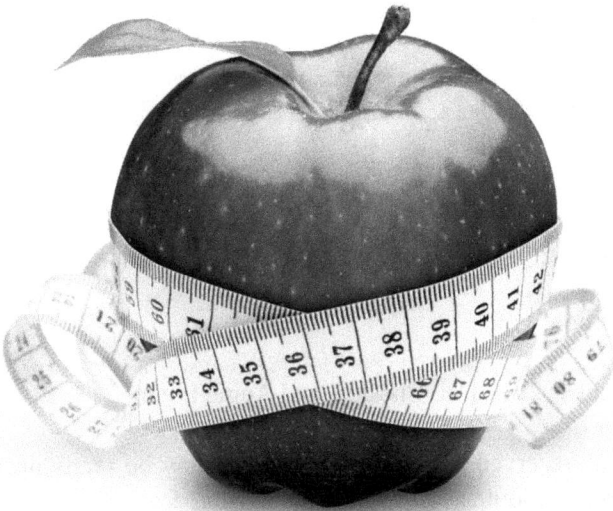

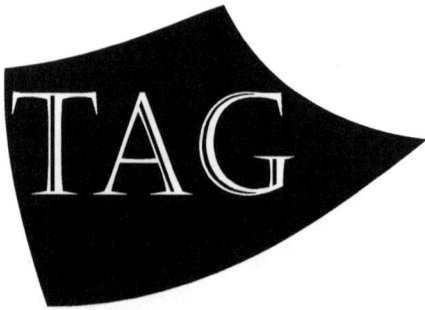

Quantity discounts are available on bulk orders.
Contact info@TAGPublishers.com for more information.

TAG Publishing, LLC
2030 S. Milam
Amarillo, TX 79109
www.TAGPublishers.com
Office (806) 373-0114
Fax (806) 373-4004
info@TAGPublishers.com

ISBN: 978-1-934606-40-7

First Edition

Release

◆ ◆ ◆

The Simple Success Solution For
Real and **Permanent** Weight Loss

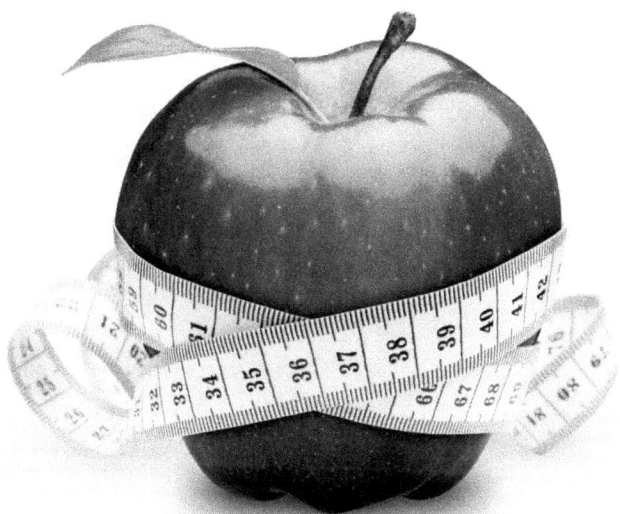

Deb Cheslow
& Angie Flynn

Contents

Contents

Acknowledgements

We are filled with gratitude for all the wonderful people who contributed to this book. It is truly the manifestation of a dream and it would not have been possible without the collaborative efforts of so many people.

First and foremost, we thank our wonderful, patient children – Erin, Nicki and Josh – who sacrificed time and attention with grace and understanding as we pushed to meet unrealistic, self-imposed deadlines. You are without a doubt our greatest creations and we love you all so very much!

We extend heartfelt gratitude to our mentor, Bob Proctor, for all his wisdom and his willingness and eagerness to unselfishly share his knowledge. You absolutely changed our lives, Bob - a debt we can never repay!

To our National Sales Director, Barry Ward. Your input into the Spirit section of this book along with your assistance during the editing process was invaluable and took the content to an entirely new level! And to our Executive Marketing Director, Freddie Smith. Thanks for being our biggest cheerleader and such an eager publicist!! We are so grateful to work with such a creative, collaborative team each and every day!

To our publisher, Dee Burks, at TAG Publishing. Thanks for being such an amazing person to work with. Your patience with us and your guidance through the process have been wonderful. We look forward to working with you for a long time to come!

To our parents, Charles and Jean Myers, and Angelo and Alice LoMascolo. Your loving upbringing and unwavering support mean more to us than you will ever know.

To all our friends in our new hometown of Port Orange, Florida – especially our friends in the Port Orange/South Daytona Chamber of Commerce and Leads III. Thank you all for the enthusiastic welcome you gave us when we arrived on the scene and for your support of our business – you can never know how much we appreciate you!

Deb Cheslow & Angie Flynn

Foreward

I have had the pleasure of knowing Deb Cheslow and Angie Flynn for well over a decade, both as patients in my practice and socially through our mutual affinity for the martial arts. I enjoy their friendship and mentorship very much. I can only imagine Deb's surprise those many years ago when she came to my office for a consultation and saw me – one of her karate students- walk through the door as the physician. The fact is that Deb did have considerable health challenges when she came to see me, among them restless leg syndrome, hypothyroidism and osteopenia. I have had the pleasure of working with thousands of patients during my career, but it is rare to encounter an individual as self-aware or as determined to overcome challenges as Deb Cheslow.

In 2008 Deb sought my assistance in weaning herself off the thyroid medication she had been taking since her partial thyroidectomy in 1997. Deb was convinced that with her diet, exercise and imagery she had resolved her hypothyroidism and wanted me to monitor her thyroid values while she tapered her medication. Much to my amazement her thyroid labs became normal and she even resolved her osteopenia and restless leg syndrome.

Deb and Angie are very physically and mentally tough women. They have endured hardship and difficult circumstances and have come out on top. They both perform at incredibly high levels athletically, but also have enviable lipid or cholesterol panels for women in their late 40's. Furthermore, these are two women that very much practice what they preach. You will not hear them espousing a set of principles and then find that they are living contrary to them. *Release* offers sound nutritional and fitness advice with the key component of training the mind to see and believe the desired result. I have witnessed both Deb and Angie's approach to fitness and nutrition firsthand over the years and I believe they have a formula for success for the individual who is willing to apply the concepts they teach.

-Robert J Young, MD

Preface

A Note from Deb and Angie

Believe... and your belief will help create the fact.
–William James

This book is about belief and one very basic question: "Do you BELIEVE that you can create a strong, fit, healthy body that you love?" Do you believe it is possible and that you can do it? Because if you don't, you may as well put this book back on the shelf or return it to wherever you bought it and get your money back. If you don't believe it's possible it will never happen. But you must have an INKLING of belief that you can do it or you wouldn't have this book in your hands now would you? If you didn't have some measure of belief you wouldn't have collected a library of diet and exercise books at home over the years as you searched for that illusive missing piece in the weight control puzzle that would FINALLY make it all work for you. Are we right? We are here to tell you that you have the ability to do incredible things in every area of your life, but you have to believe it yourself. Even the Bible tells us *"...if you have faith the size of a mustard seed, you will say to this mountain, 'Move from here to there,' and it will move; and nothing will be impossible to you." (Matthew 17:20).* All science and all religion tell us that we all have immense reservoirs of talent and ability within us – we just have to learn how to tap into them. And THAT begins with BELIEF!!

We decided to title this book *Release* because that's what you want to do with excess weight – you want to RELEASE it – let it go – FOREVER!! You shouldn't say that you want to "*LOSE*" 15 pounds because you have been programmed all your life to FIND whatever you LOSE and we don't know about you, but we don't want any of these pounds of blubber back – EVER!! We have no intention of finding them again.

The *Release* Plan is designed to work for everyone. It offers options for people at every point along the weight control spectrum. If you weigh 400 pounds and have done little more for exercise for the past 10 years than walk to the kitchen to get your next snack, then *Release* is for you – it gives you a place to start, without overwhelming you. If you are a veteran "gym rat" who makes it your business to study the latest trends in diet and exercise, then *Release* is also for you – it refreshes you on the basics, and shows you how to take your nutrition and fitness to the next level.

You know, perception is a very interesting thing. Angie actually found the program Deb used initially to begin her weight release journey a couple of years before Deb was introduced to it, but dismissed it because of her perception about weight lifting. "I thought weightlifting was fine for men, but that women who lifted looked 'lumpy' and freakish. It was a complete misperception of fact. I had the answer in my hands, but I was so freaked out about the idea of lifting weights at a gym that I 'threw the baby out with the bath water.' " Likewise, Deb dismissed many a book on the subject of weight control or exercise because they seemed too "elementary" on the surface, even though they may have offered her great insight. It was important to us as we were writing *Release* to take all levels into account and provide great value to all.

But here's the deal, we are offering you the paint, the paintbrush and the canvas, but the picture you choose to paint is entirely up to you. We can absolutely guarantee that if you do exactly what we say in this book, you will absolutely achieve your ideal weight and create a body that looks, feels and performs magnificently. However, half-hearted efforts produce half-hearted results. If you do everything except "that" (whatever "that" is) because it makes you uncomfortable or everything in chapter 1; 3 of the 5 things in Chapter 2; eat 4 meals instead of 6; exercise only 1 day per week and have 3 free days per week, well then, don't expect much!

It's important that you know that we are NOT doctors, we do NOT have degrees or certifications in nutrition, exercise physiology, or psychology. We do NOT spend hours each day in the gym or the kitchen. We have lives – very busy lives. We are partners, moms, homemakers and we run a very active, successful business. We generally work between 10-12 hours per day – sometimes a lot more.

We tell you this not to impress you, but to impress upon you that we're just regular people – we have to fit it all into 24 hours each day just the same as you. We got sick and tired of being sick and tired so we researched and we experimented and we sought help from people who did know what they were doing and we figured it all out. If we can do it, YOU can do it – there is no doubt about it!!

Deb Cheslow & Angie Flynn

Introduction

Everyone wants a magic bullet to fix their problems, but
nobody believes in magic.
–The Mad Hatter, Once Upon A Time

Angie's Story

Release is the realization of a dream that started as one of
those pesky, niggling ideas that just won't leave you alone. I hired
Deb as my "life coach" in early 2010. She immediately started
introducing me to the idea that you become what you think
about and that your thoughts are the key to creating the future
that you want. It was so simple and so obvious once I had that
awareness, and I quickly realized that I had been spending the past
4 decades of my life expending an incredible amount of perfect
thought energy on creating exactly what I DIDN'T want – and
was surprised when I kept receiving more and more of it!! One
area of my life that I continually struggled with was my weight.
I was never truly FAT – at my heaviest (non-pregnant) point I
weighed 183 lbs, which was too heavy for my 5'5" frame, but not
morbidly obese by a long shot. I was obsessed with dieting. I had a
whole collection of diet books and I read them over and over again
looking for the missing piece of the puzzle that would make the
weight simply fall off. I wasn't really looking for a "magic bullet"
– I was willing to do the work, but I wanted a plan that actually
did WORK!! It was shortly after I started working with Deb that
I realized that, all of a sudden, I was shrinking. Yes, I was eating
better and I was working out more, but I had done all that before
– something was different this time. The weight was falling off
so fast that my family started to worry that something might be
wrong with me. I went from a size 12 to a size 8 in a little over
2 months. Muscles started to appear. My stamina was incredible.
What was the difference? One evening I started brainstorming
what was happening to me with Deb and the answer presented
itself. It wasn't the *process* that was so different, but rather that
I was different. Rather than focusing on the imperfections that
I saw in the mirror, I had begun to visualize myself at my "ideal

weight" – even though I had no clue what that NUMBER actually was. I would close my eyes and see myself step up onto the scale and look down and see the perfect weight staring back at me in all of its digital glory. The more I did this, the easier I found it to get up early to exercise, to get in an extra karate class at night, to make the proper food choices throughout the day. My self-image – that picture of myself that I carry around inside my mind – was shifting and as it did my physical body was shifting to match it.

So, back to the idea for the book... Deb and I had just sent the manuscript of *The Simple Success Solution* to editing in August, 2010 and one day I was just pondering how on earth I managed to change from an overweight, unhappy, functional alcoholic who was a financially, emotionally and otherwise broken mess, to a person who was financially free, mentally and physically healthy and deliriously happy. I had literally transformed into a person who absolutely jumped out of bed every morning excited about life and what was in store for me that day - in just a few short months – how does that happen? And then this little voice started whispering in my ear that our next book needed to be about the mind-body-spirit connection in weight control. There were a million different books out there that went into excruciating detail about the "body" part and a few that delved into the "spirit" side of things, but I had never read a "diet" book that spent any serious time on the connection between weight and self image – how the mind controls the body. It was the missing piece!! I started talking to Deb about writing a book on the subject and she was all for it, but then I kept dismissing the idea because who was I to present myself as an authority on weight control? I didn't have any degrees or credentials that supported such a lofty vision, so I let the dream go. However, as most worthy ideals do, the idea just wouldn't leave me alone. It would pop up every so often and I would noodle on it for a while, and talk to Deb about it and she would tell me it was a great idea and then I'd dismiss it again as silliness. This went on until late 2011. The voice was back telling me that I had an important book locked inside me and it was my responsibility to share it. Again, I brought up the subject to Deb and she turned and looked at me and said, "Angie, can we write the damned book already? I've been listening to you talk about it for over a year now… LET'S WRITE THE BOOK!!" And so, we wrote the book…

As we outlined it, it was clear that there needed to be separate sections that addressed "Mind," "Body," and "Spirit," but it still seemed incomplete. My favorite weight control books were ones that had stories from people who had made the program work – I loved reading about their successes, but I always wondered how many times they fell off the wagon on their journey? Did they ever succumb to potato chips and chocolate cake? Did they ever wake up and say "Oh God NO, not today?" Were they human? So, I decided that *Release* needed to follow someone through the process of releasing their extra weight. The last half of 2011 was incredibly busy and stressful for our business and our family and I had put on a few pounds that I wasn't terribly happy with, so who better to use as a case study than myself. The picture at the left was

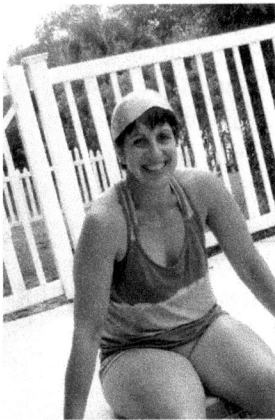

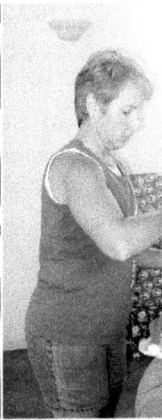

taken on August 7, 2011. Although, I don't have many pictures of myself – I'm usually happily behind the camera - you can see that I'm "bottom heavy" here. The picture on the right was taken on Christmas Eve, 2011 and I weighed 158 lbs. I was NOT happy about it! On January 2, 2012 I started "releasing!" I committed to give readers the entire story – the good, the bad, the ugly, the compromises, the justifications, the triumphs and the failures on the road to my ideal weight. There are lots of stories in this book and a lot of places where I tripped and fell along the way. The biggest lesson I learned was that the number on the scale does not define who I am or what I am worth as a person. This is a lifestyle for me – a journey that I will continue and you can follow along with me and get all of the glorious (and sometimes ugly) detail week by week and month by month at *MyReleasePlan.com.*

Deb's Story

My story is quite different from Angie's. I have always lived what others might call a "charmed life." If I set my sights on a goal at any point in my life I achieved it, despite the odds against success. I never had a weight problem as a child – I was very active and participated on a number of sports teams, including softball, volleyball and basketball throughout high school. My diet consisted of, well, crap - pop-tarts for breakfast, pepperoni and ketchup sandwiches and Twinkies for lunch, a hot dog from the local convenience store on the way home from practice, whatever Mom fixed for dinner and a big bowl of ice cream or a milkshake before bed. I have to cringe when I think about what I was putting in my body back then. My exercise regimen consisted of whatever after-school team practice was scheduled for the day, but I wasn't a gym rat, I didn't do any strength training in any organized consistent manner and I wasn't interested in aerobics classes. I was blessed with a naturally thin, athletic physique. The picture to the left was snapped in 1983 just after I graduated from high school – natural 6-pack abs, ah those were the days!!!

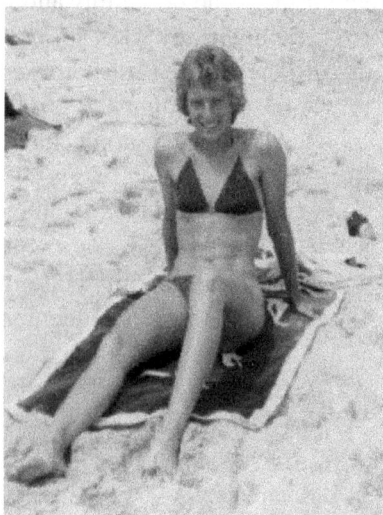

In college I was in the Air Force Corps of Cadets and after school sports practice was replaced by a lot of stress, late night study sessions and military drills – hardly physically taxing - but I kept eating the way I always had and over the course of my Freshman year I gained 15 lbs. For the first time in my life I started dabbling in dieting. I made a conscious decision to "eat right." Now, keep in mind, all that meant for me was not eating bagels and pizza before bed and not eating unlimited portions at the dining hall, or running across the street to the fast food places whenever I wanted something. It did not at all mean "healthy" eating.

One of my friends in the dorm was on a high protein, low carb diet and I messed around with that, but not strictly. For the first time in my life I was aware of what I was eating and was trying to control it. By the time I graduated I was back down to 123 lbs. My activity dramatically increased during my junior and senior year – there was a lot more physical training involved and I was very active. I had also taken up running during this time. However, looking back, it is obvious to me that the main reason I didn't gain a substantial amount of weight was because I didn't give any energy to it. In my mind I was 118 lbs and in great shape and so even though there was a momentary blip during my freshman year, I behaved in ways that were consistent with being 118 lbs.

I graduated from college in June, 1987 and didn't report to the Air Force until March of the following year. During that time I really concentrated on "getting in shape" – I joined a gym, lifted weights for the first time, and went on long bike rides. It was the first time I was exercising for the sake of exercise (as opposed to "training" for something) and I really got hooked on it. I added muscle to my body during this time and although I still weighed 123 lbs, I was smaller in size than I had ever been.

After reporting to the Air Force, life took on an incredible momentum – pilot training, instructor pilot training and then actually teaching other airmen to fly. I was very active, but there was no real time in my day for a structured exercise plan. I was always aware of what I was eating, and in my mind I was controlling my portions, but I was still eating CRAP and lots of calories, yet I stayed right at 123 lbs. That was my self-image and it didn't matter how many KFC chicken and biscuits or potato skins, or bags of sun chips I ate, I stayed right at 123 lbs. I loved my job, I jumped out of bed every morning to do what I was doing, and was always a tad incredulous when money showed up in my bank account twice per month – I was actually getting PAID to have fun all day long. I was a ridiculously happy person – there was no energy given to anything negative, so good things just kept showing up in my life, including meeting and marrying the man of my dreams.

Deb Cheslow & Angie Flynn

Shortly after we got married, I got pregnant with daughter #1. It was a textbook pregnancy, during which I gained 30 lbs (I was always kind of proud of the fact that even at the height of my pregnancy, I never topped the Air Force weight maximum for a non-pregnant person). After Erin was born, I found myself back at 123 pounds in record time. 12 months later I was pregnant with baby #2 and found myself faced with a huge decision. The Air Force re-assigned me to a position that would have taken me away from my husband and children for extended periods of time. This was NOT an option for me. I was already having a really difficult time with the idea of "someone else" raising my kids – we had a great nanny, but she wasn't ME! I decided to separate from the Air Force, to stay at home with my daughters and be a stay-at-home-mom. It was very interesting – I LOVED being with my girls, but I found that I no longer jumped out of bed in the morning. I had gained the same 30 pounds during my second pregnancy as with my first, but I couldn't seem to get rid of it all afterwards. I focused on exercise, but it seemed like nothing I did worked.

For the next 5 years I tried every diet under the sun – I would do it religiously (almost to the point of obsessive) for 60 days. I was focusing on losing weight but nothing was working. My weight was either staying stable or creeping up. I wasn't morbidly obese by any stretch – at my heaviest I was wearing a size 10, but I wanted my size 6 body back!! I was getting desperate – even to the point of popping "diet pills." All I focused on was "there has to be a way to lose these 10 lbs!" But nothing I tried was working.

Then one day I was talking with one of my daughter's pre-school teachers and she introduced me to a new exercise and nutrition program and she suggested we do it together. Something about the way she was talking about it intrigued me. I researched it during a trip and it sparked something in me – it made sense to me and I knew it was the answer. The fact that is was based on both strength training and cardiovascular conditioning workouts re-ignited what I had started back when I was in between college and the Air Force. I KNEW it was the answer. I BELIEVED it and all my OCD tendencies were funneled into doing this program perfectly for 90 days. I got my husband on the bandwagon and I pushed myself hard at every workout. I measured my portions of food obsessively. I filled out every menu plan, every workout sheet. After 90 days, it very much became a part of who I was – it became habitual. Plus I had two great accountability partners – my husband and my friend who introduced me to the program.

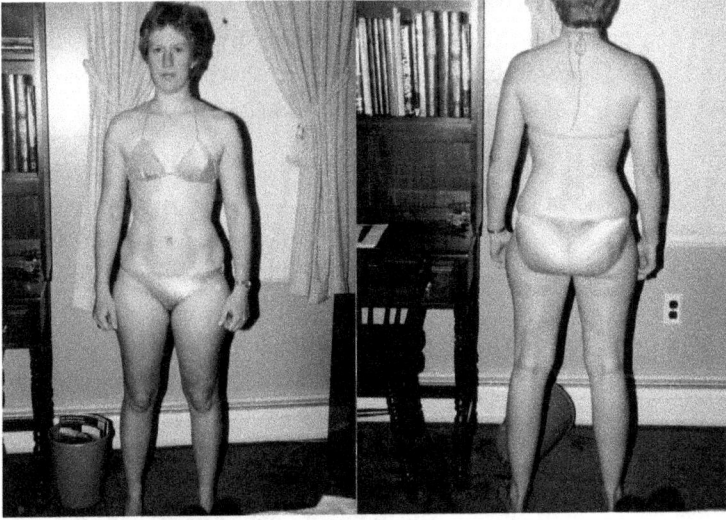

August, 2000

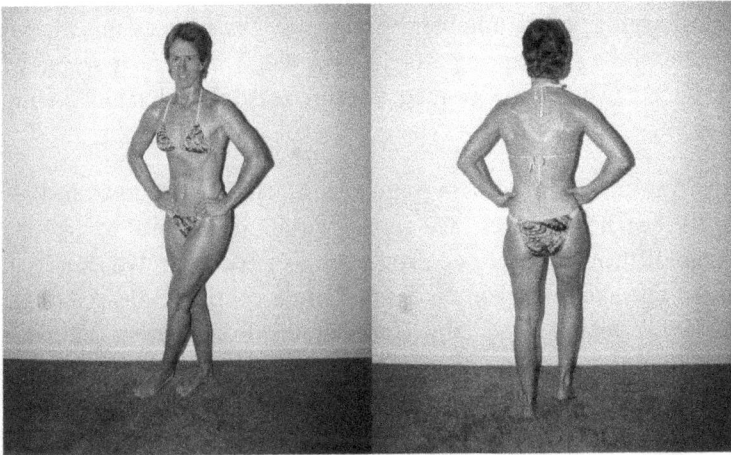

November, 2000 (after 90 days)

After 90 days on the program, I had gained a great deal of muscle and released a lot of fat and weighed 127 lbs. Although not the 123 lbs I was in college, I was actually smaller, looked better and was proud of the body I had built. But then a funny thing happened over the next few years. I found that every spring I was gaining 3-4 lbs and my weight average was creeping up at the rate of about a pound per year. I saw it happening and I was just exasperated. I would step up the exercise and cut my meals to the bare core (I never "restricted," but I went back to basics), doing every part of the program obsessively and yet every spring my weight would be up 3-4lbs.

In 2004 I coached a friend through my eating and exercise plan – he couldn't afford to buy the supplements that I used and he couldn't afford a gym membership, but he made all it work on his farm (filling milk jugs with sand and getting creative with strength training) and he transformed. One day at karate we were talking and I had a huge A-HA moment. I was talking about how I just couldn't seem to get back to 127 lbs and he said "Who cares what the scale says if you like what you look like." And although I KNEW that and had even said it to people I had coached through the program, I had never applied it to myself. The moment I gave myself permission to focus on what I loved about my body and to forget about what the scale said, I kept getting more of what I loved – my body continued transforming and getting better and better. Once I leapt this mental hurdle, the annual spring weight gain didn't happen. It seemed I could eat whatever I wanted (within reason) and maintain my weight.

A case in point, back in August, 2010, Angie and I took the kids to the beach for a week. We very purposefully planned to take the week off from a structured eating and exercise plan. We exercised if we felt like it (which we did on only a couple of days) and we ate/drank what we wanted, which included frozen drinks and wine every afternoon, eating out at a variety of restaurants and just ENJOYING ourselves without limitation – it was a very abundant week!! But even with the week off, both Angie and I came back from vacation without gaining an ounce – Angie actually released a pound while on vacation!

Fast forward to Summer, 2011... I had tested for my 2nd degree black belt in karate the year before and my instructor had essentially told me he had taken me as far as he could. Although I would continue to test for more advanced belts, I wouldn't be truly "challenged" to any great extent from here on. That was tough to take – karate was such a huge part of my motivation – preparing for tests and training to be better and stronger. Now there was no goal. I kept going through the motions for Angie – she had very ambitious physical goals and I wanted to support her in them - but you can't live for someone else's goals; there is no inspiration in that, regardless of how much you love the other person. I found myself justifying skipping workouts, I ate too much of the wrong kinds of foods. All of my energy and focus was on the move to Florida and on building our business in our new hometown. Well, what you give energy to grows and what you ignore dies. I was not giving any mental energy to having an ideal body so I gained some weight, I felt awful, I was tired all the time and I was just DONE!

On January 1, 2012, Angie and I agreed to go back to the basics. Eating correctly and working out six days per week were not optional; they were part of our lifestyle and would not be sacrificed. I re-focused on being in fantastic shape and looking great, not on what the scale said. We were writing this book and there is nothing more important than for me to be in integrity – practicing what I preach! I feel a great sense of purpose again and life is very good!

So, how did 90 days on the *Release* Plan work out for us? Better than we ever hoped - stay tuned for our results and the amazing lessons we learned along the way.

Deb Cheslow & Angie Flynn

Mind

Whatever the mind can conceive and believe, it can achieve.
–Napoleon Hill

Deb Cheslow & Angie Flynn

CHAPTER ONE

THE MISSING PIECE

Why is this "mind stuff" important?

Well, it's really not unless you want to ensure that your plan is successful. One of the main forces behind our desire to write this book sprung from our awareness that there are thousands of books on the market (maybe hundreds of thousands) that profess to show you a path to permanent weight release and fitness. They give the reader a step-by step plan for achieving a healthier body, but we have not come across ONE that addresses the missing piece of the puzzle – the fact that the physical transformation begins on the *inside* long before the decision to release the weight is made – it begins with the self-image of the person who is executing the plan – in this case, YOU!

Everyone has a unique self-image – no two are alike, so no one cookie-cutter weight release program will work for every person in the same way. The first thing that has to happen in order for you to change the behavior that has brought you to where you are is to understand WHY you behave that way in the first place. And to understand that it is critical that you understand a bit about how the mind works, so stick with us!! This section of the book is far more important than the diet and exercise part (although that is important too)- it's the missing piece in the puzzle of weight control (and everything else in your life as well).

Your Glorious Mind

Our minds hold the key to an unlimited potential within each of us, yet the vast majority of people fail to tap into this powerful force. Why is that? Well, one big problem is that far too many people have no idea what "*MIND*" is. Very often when we ask people what they think of when they hear the word "mind", they say "brain." MOST people use the terms "mind" and "brain" interchangeably. But nothing could be farther from the truth - they are very different and distinct. We like to describe the brain as the radio and the mind as the music. The music is transmitted through the radio, it doesn't originate from it. Much in the same manner the brain is the biological organ inside the skull and our thoughts don't originate from it. The brain is on the physical plane – you can see it, measure it, and touch it (although that would be gross). Mind, however, is movement – it's on the spiritual plane. Mind is an activity found in every cell of our being. Think about it for a minute, it is rumored that Albert Einstein's brain is housed in a jar in a laboratory somewhere in New Jersey, but it's of absolutely no use to anyone (other than those who may have studied it's anatomy and structure) because Einstein's MIND isn't with it any longer. The brain is a physical organ and its functions include muscle control and coordination, sensory reception and integration, and speech – it's an electrical switching station. The brain is a part of our central nervous system while the mind controls the higher functions, such as memory, reason, and thought. The mind is the description of our conceptualization of what we think, analyze, and project.

When we are talking about the mind, we first need to distinguish between its two separate and distinct facets, which are the **Conscious** mind and the **Subconscious** mind.

When we are working with our clients, we start by making the distinction between the mind and the brain, but we have to add a visual image of what the mind "looks" like. See, when you and I think, we literally think in pictures. And the clearer the picture we have of something, the more order and the less fear, doubt, and confusion we experience. Think about it, if we ask you to think of your car, or your home, a picture or an image of your car or your home will flash on the screen of your mind. Not your mom's car, or your friend's car or the letters C-A-R, but **your** car. And the thing is, this is working all the time, whether you want it to or not. As human beings we think in pictures – PERIOD. Let us prove it to you. Right now, no matter what you do, DON'T think about a pink elephant. Did you see a picture of a massive pink thing with big ears and a long nose flash across your mind? We're willing to bet so. It is true: we think in pictures. Mind is the screen on which those pictures pop up when we ask you to think of your car or home, or the pink elephant. When we ask our clients to visualize what the mind looks like, most of them envision a picture of a brain. Our mind looks nothing like the giant head of cauliflower we've all seen in encyclopedias or in 7th grade science class. Because our mind is not on the physical plane, no one has ever seen it – and no one ever will - there is no picture. But yet, as human beings, we think in pictures so for us to have a true understanding of the mind, we must have a clear mental picture to work with. No picture leads to confusion. So, we need a picture to work with.

In 1934, Dr. Thurman Fleet, chiropractor and founder of the Concept Therapy Institute, was working with his patients to literally heal themselves of ailments by "thinking" themselves healthy. However, he kept running up against this same roadblock when discussing the mind's role in healing the body with them. They had no visual frame of reference for the concept of "mind." Dr. Fleet decided that since our thoughts are visual, we need a picture of our mind. As a result of his decision, a very simple yet profound tool known as the "Stick Person" emerged. Dr. Fleet's drawing brings order and understanding to our mind and is a fantastic tool we can use to explain how our thoughts affect how we see ourselves, and ultimately determine our results. It makes absolutely no difference that Dr. Fleet actually made up the picture – as long as we can associate an image with a concept we can develop understanding and application. So now, let's examine the following image of the Stick Person.

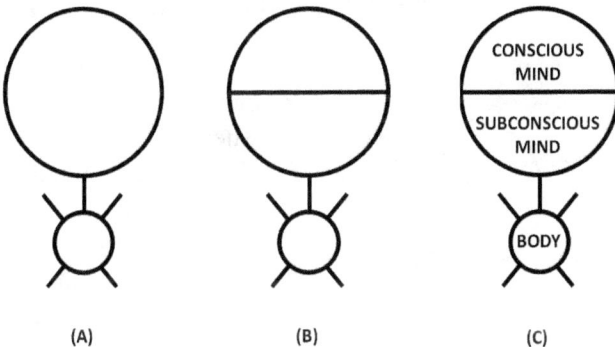

(A)   (B)   (C)

We start with a version of the stick figure person that every one of us drew a million times in kindergarten, only in this version the head is purposely drawn disproportionately larger than the body (A). This is because the mind is the dominant force in our lives, not the body; the body is merely an instrument of the mind; that is, the body carries out the "commands" it receives from the mind. To further illustrate our stickperson, we add a horizontal line bisecting the head into two halves (B). The top half of the head represents the Conscious Mind, or our *thinking* mind and the lower half represents the Subconscious Mind, or our *emotional* mind (C). Thoughts (in our conscious mind) cause us to experience feelings (in our subconscious mind), which drive the body into action, which in turn leads us to manifest the results we are getting in our lives. What we want you to start understanding is that our results are ultimately driven by our thoughts, so if you can change your thoughts to produce different feelings to drive your body into different actions, you cannot fail to achieve different results.

In order for us to have healthy thoughts and release our old outdated thoughts, we must have a clear and concise comprehension of how our mind works. Don't get nervous here, we're not talking psychiatry or psychology; this is not complicated stuff – it's just that we've never been taught this information before. But with a very elementary understanding of how our mind functions, we have the ability to tap into an immense power that lies largely dormant within each of us. Let's take our Stick Person apart piece by piece and see what's really going on here.

The Conscious Mind

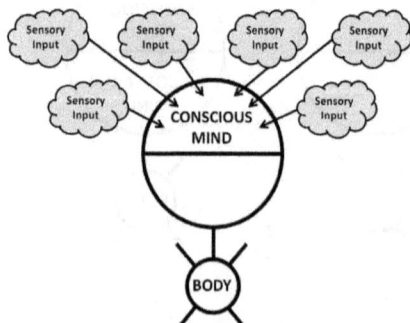

Our Conscious Mind is our thinking mind. This is where our free will resides. The conscious mind has the ability to accept or reject any idea introduced to it. Our five senses—sight, hearing taste, touch, and smell are continually pumping in sensory inputs and stimuli from our outside environment. The conscious mind reads and interprets the inputs received from our physical senses. Because we think in pictures, any time one or all of our five senses is triggered we immediately create a picture in our mind. This is much like a satellite dish that transmits signals to your television set or a cell phone tower that transmits signals to your phone. Think of the conscious mind as the highway that all this external information travels on to enter your subconscious mind. Various feelings occur depending on the different interpretations we give to these external stimuli. For instance, does the smell of a certain perfume bring back memories of your grandmother? Or does the taste of a cherry snow cone remind you of the beach or summer afternoons spent at the swimming pool as a child? As these sensory inputs are received, your conscious mind has the power to accept or reject the thoughts associated with them. If the conscious mind chooses to accept the thoughts, the subconscious mind has no choice but to generate the feelings triggered by those thoughts.

Everything on the physical plane is a manifestation of our thought. Everything in your awareness—everything you see that is manmade—it all started as a thought. The clothes you are wearing, the computer you sneak a peek at Facebook on, the chair you are sitting on, the house you live in, the cell phone your spouse just texted you on - EVERYTHING begins in thought, as someone's unrealistic fantasy. You have to understand that all of your bodily experiences are an expression of your mind and if you don't truly believe that you won't see the results you want.

The Subconscious Mind

As mentioned before, the subconscious mind has no ability to reject any idea or thought impressed upon it; it simply must accept every suggestion made to it—it is your emotional or feeling mind. By assembling various facts, your conscious mind draws conclusions which generate emotions and feelings, in your subconscious mind. For example, if you step on the scales for your weekly weigh-in and you see that you have released 4 pounds, your conscious mind processes that sensory input and impresses the information on your subconscious mind. You can't help the FEELINGS that well up inside you – happiness that you are closer to your goal, pride in your accomplishment, exhilaration that your body is becoming thinner, etc. Likewise, if at that same weigh-in you discover that you have gained 4 pounds that week you can't help the feelings that are generated – disappointment, failure, self-deprecation, etc. The thoughts in our conscious mind cause feelings/emotional response in our subconscious mind. Each thought you think and accept is impressed upon the subconscious part of your mind and it can't tell the difference between what is real and what is imagined; it accepts everything as fact.

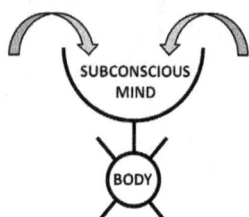

Let's take this a step further. When you were born you didn't have a conscious mind – your conscious faculties don't develop for several years. So as a baby, you were essentially like the picture at the left. Your subconscious mind was WIDE OPEN and took in everything it heard going on around you. For the first few years of life babies are like little sponges soaking in every sensory input they receive from their parents, their grandparents, their brothers and sisters, their babysitters, the television and radio, etc., right into their subconscious mind. Think about how quickly we learn to speak our native language. It's because there are no conscious faculties to get in our way – we just learn it. It's the same with learning how to walk – we don't know anything about "self-imposed limitations," so we keep trying until one day we're walking. Think about how HARD some of the things you learned to do as a small child are – how IMPOSSIBLE they are for many adults (have you ever tried to become fluent in another language as an adult or had to learn to walk or talk all over again after some traumatic injury?) – think about all we are capable of if we can just get out of our own way!!!

So, as a baby and a small child you were taking this information from your external environment into your subconscious mind like a vacuum; it sucked in every word, thought, or action it came into contact with, and stored it all as truth. Your subconscious mind is a storage unit for all that has happened in your life. It stores your beliefs which include your emotional connections to the past. We think of it as a scrapbook containing all of our past experiences. What you feel, think, or do forms the basis of your experiences, which are stored in the form of underlying impressions in the subconscious mind. This is why it is so difficult to release your old, self-destructive thoughts or defeating behaviors. What was going on around you when you were a child? What kind of information was your subconscious mind sucking in about your weight? Your body? How you looked?

*Angie's Story: When I was a child I was chunky – never FAT, but stocky – solid. My sister, on the other hand, was a beanpole – very thin, very small boned. My family always compared us – not in a mean-spirited sort of way, but the comparison was stark. I was chubby and she was thin, I had an olive complexion, dark eyes and black hair (favoring our Sicilian ancestors) and she was very fair with blonde hair and blue eyes (favoring our Northern Italian relatives). My mother, who was a veteran in the dieting arena, tried everything she could to help me lose weight. I never really thought about it until the summer after 7th grade when she enrolled me in a study that the university's psychology department was conducting on "obese children." **OBESE** children... Gosh, I can still see the words on that sign as we went to check in on that first day – it still makes me feel sick to my stomach. It was an emotional impact moment for me. I remember having to get on the scales and then do a bunch of exercises and talk about what I ate. We were sent home with a diet plan and workout charts and I had to go back every week all summer and get weighed and measured. It was humiliating and embarrassing and I HATED it. What those 12 weeks implanted deeply into my subconscious mind was that I was an obese child – even though at 5'2" tall I weighed 115 lbs – hardly obese. I spent the next 30+ years in a constant battle with my self-image and my weight bounced up and down over and over again – I've lost and gained HUNDREDS of pounds and in the end,*

I just kept getting bigger and bigger. I don't blame my mother – she didn't know what was happening - she was just trying to help me develop healthy eating and exercise habits, but the damage was done nonetheless.

And that's the point in most cases – the people who "programmed" you when you were a child thought they were doing the very best for you. They loved you and wanted you to be the most fabulous version of you possible, but they were unaware of what was happening. Any image or pattern of images that is repeatedly impressed upon your subconscious mind becomes part of your habitual patterns. A habit is something you do without conscious thought – like brushing your teeth (do you actually focus on each stroke of the toothbrush or do you think about what you need to do once you get to the office or about what you'll have for dinner) or driving a car (can you imagine what would happen if you had to consciously think about all the steps you needed to take to stop a car as you approach a stop light). A *collection of habits* is known as a *paradigm*. Paradigms develop as expectations or assumptions about what and how things should be done. And there are as many different paradigms as there are people – no two are exactly alike, because the experiences of no two people are exactly alike. It is that collection of paradigms that determines your self-image – what you believe you are capable of, what you deserve, and yes, whether you are thin or fat.

Repeated Image ➜ Habit ➜ Paradigm
(Collection of Habits) ➜ Self-Image

The way your self-image operates can be compared to a thermostat in your home. You set the thermostat to keep the house at a nice, comfortable 70°F. It doesn't really matter what the temperature is outside, the house stays at 70°. We live in Florida and it can get brutally hot outside during the day. Let's say our son goes outside to play and leaves the front door standing open. The heat from the outside begins to raise the temperature inside. As soon as the temperature goes above 70°, the thermostat takes over and causes the air conditioning system to turn on. Cool air begins blowing through the duct work and into the rooms until the temperature in the house comes back down to 70°. The only thing we need to do is close the front door!

Your self-image regarding your weight, your income level, your relationships, your career – pretty much everything in your life – operates in a very similar fashion. Using the example of weight control: You decide you want to release the excess weight on your body, so you start a new nutrition and fitness program (a "diet") and you follow it to the letter for the first week. You eat exactly the way the plan prescribes and you work out when and how the plan tells you to and you get to the end of the week and get on the scales and see you have indeed reduced your weight by a few pounds. You may go along like this for weeks or months and continue to drop weight, but if you haven't addressed your self-image – if you haven't changed the thermostat - you will very subtly begin to sabotage your progress. Maybe you justify eating something that is not on your meal plan because you've been so good for so long – surely just this one time won't hurt anything, and then that one time becomes an all day binge or the one day becomes a whole week. Or, perhaps you justify a "cheat" and then beat yourself up because you were weak. Then you convince yourself that you've blown your diet, so you may as well just quit and start over again on Monday. Slowly but surely your weight begins to climb and in the sum total of things you end up back where you started or with a few extra pounds added in just for good measure. Does that sound familiar?

Have you ever wondered why there seems to be a certain weight that you find incredibly easy to maintain? It doesn't matter what you eat (or don't eat), you just seem to stay at that weight? That "set point" is the weight that is in complete alignment with your self-image, your thermostat setting, and you will always come back to it automatically.

Angie's Story: As we were writing this book, I was actually using the program to release the extra weight I was carrying around. I could see physical changes on my body, but every Saturday morning my weight would be exactly the same as it had been the previous week – the scales just wouldn't budge! It was only once I covered up the scale readout with a picture of my goal weight and let Deb check the actual weight each Saturday morning (she didn't tell me what the number was, she just logged it) that the weight started to drop. It was as if my mind was keeping me stuck on a certain number.

It is essential that you use the tools that are in this section to begin to reprogram your self-image if you ever want to achieve permanent weight release.

Deepak Chopra and Wayne Dyer often quote a study that concludes that our minds are bombarded by an average of 65,000 thoughts per day. Yet the studies also show that the human brain only processes between 2,500 and 3,500 of those thoughts per day, each ranging from 12-14 seconds long. According to these same studies, the more focused you are on something the fewer thoughts you will actually process each day. For instance, elite athletes only process an average of 1,500 thoughts per day because they are so focused on what they are doing in any given moment. Why is it that over 99% of the thoughts that invade our minds each day just "bounce off" and we don't even realize it? It goes back to the paradigms and the self image that reside in our subconscious mind – they actually set up a "filter" around our conscious mind which only allows thoughts that are consistent with our paradigms and our beliefs to pass through.

Let's ponder this for a moment. Have you ever had a female friend who seems to stay effortlessly thin, regardless of what she eats or how much (or how little) she exercises? Have you ever had one of these friends get pregnant and watch them gain 30, 40, 50, even 60 lbs. during their pregnancy and yet 6 weeks after their baby is born they are back in the jeans they were wearing before they got pregnant? And yet another friend who struggles mightily with her weight every day gains the same amount of weight during a pregnancy and never seems to release it all. Why the difference? Yes, there could be differences in metabolism and body type and such that certainly may play a part, but we submit that the overriding reason for the difference is that the first friend has a thin self-image and the second friend has a fat self-image.

The filters that are set around their conscious minds are different, so they are aware of different thoughts. The first friend is absolutely aware of what she needs to do to fit back in those jeans and her thoughts (in her conscious mind) and her feelings (generated by the paradigm/self-image in her subconscious mind) are in complete harmony, so she naturally just acts in ways that are consistent with shedding the extra weight and getting back in her pre-pregnancy jeans. The other friend's filter is not letting in the thoughts that would lead her to naturally and effortlessly make the choices she needs to make to release the extra weight. Those thoughts are not in harmony with her self-image, so although she KNOWS what to do intellectually, she can't make herself DO what she knows. She may force a certain behavior for a time, but eventually the self-image wins and the weight comes back.

The logical question then is "Can I change the filter? Can I change my paradigms and my self-image?" The answer is "Of course you can!!" Just because you have one self-image today doesn't mean you can't change it! When you build big beautiful pictures of everything you want to be, do, or have, your subconscious mind has no choice but to accept these thoughts as fact. With repetition over time, you can create a new self-image and create a new *physical* reality. The process is "simple," but not necessarily easy, but don't worry we will walk you through the process, step by step and give you all kinds of tools to use to make the journey easier!!

Since your subconscious mind has no choice but to accept what you think, you have to nourish it with healthy and encouraging information. It's really no different than your physical body – if you sit on your butt on the sofa and watch the garbage that's on TV and eat potato chips all day there is no way that you are going to be either physically or mentally healthy. If you don't make a conscious effort to take control of your self-destructive thoughts,

Deb Cheslow & Angie Flynn

they'll take over and rot out the positive ones, leaving your life a crumbling mess. Your subconscious mind is incredibly powerful. Have you heard the saying "Thoughts become things?" It's so true – you think a thought in your conscious mind and impress that thought on your subconscious mind over and over again and the feelings associated with the thought move you into actions that are consistent with the thought. If you mistakenly focus on what you don't want, you will bring about those results. The subconscious mind expresses itself in your feelings which lead to your actions and behavior, and actions produce results (sorry, but you have to take action to produce results – anything else is just wishful thinking). When you string a bunch of these goal-driven actions together you can begin to see how your reality will also change. By learning to apply this knowledge to your life, you realize that you **can** have whatever you want in life.

Thoughts ➔ Feelings ➔ Actions ➔ Results

See, your paradigms are stored in your subconscious mind and are expressed through your actions. So if your parents treated you like you were stupid, stubborn, lazy or fat, you came to believe it This behavior helped to establish a paradigm and build our self-image. Paradigms are the governing belief systems that determine your success in life. And the thing about paradigms is this: they're not even YOURS! Remember the baby with the wide open subconscious mind? Who "programmed" that baby's subconscious? His or her parents, right? Well, who programmed the parents? Yep, their parents and so on and so on. Some paradigms are GENERATIONS old. You know, your authors feel that if you're going to have a paradigm that's screwing up your life, then darn it, you should have some say in the matter!

So what ARE your paradigms? Well, if you want to know what you have been thinking subconsciously, just take a look at your present results. Are you overweight? Are your brothers and/or sisters overweight? Your parents? Your grandparents? Your CHILDREN? Paradigms surrounding weight and health are some of the most common paradigms passed down through the generations (another being attitudes surrounding money).

And because of this you may be consciously aware of what is going on with the other people around you and not see that you are doing the exact same things. Here's one of Angie's examples:

Angie's Story: I grew up in a home where my mother constantly worried about her weight. She wasn't particularly overweight to start, but she always thought she needed to lose a couple of pounds so she exercised every morning only to eat ice cream and potato chips each night and cry each time she stepped on the scale. My mother's fear of being overweight was ingrained in me and still haunts me today. As a child I remember saying to myself, "I will not live this way when I grow up." But, jump ahead twenty years and there I was a few pounds overweight, constantly trying to find a way to lose them. I would work so hard during the day— exercising, practicing discipline and self-control only to fall apart at night, eating—guess what—ice cream and potato chips— just like Mom! How much of an effect do you think my upbringing had to do with this scenario? And all that time I had no idea what my subconscious conditioning was making me do!

The Body

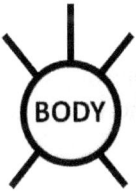

The body is the smallest part of the Stick Person. It is drawn this way to illustrate the concept that your physical body is merely an instrument of the mind and is your outward physical manifestation to the world. Although it may not seem like it, your body is fairly insignificant and weak when compared to your mind. However, without the body there can be no action, and therefore, no results. Before you can CREATE what you want in your life you must DECIDE what you want and then you must take ACTION toward your goal EVERY DAY!! It would be so great if we could just close our eyes tight and clasp our hands and think "125 lbs, 125 lbs, 125 lbs" and jump on the scales and be at our ideal weight, but that's not how it works

Would you agree that you KNOW how to release the excess weight you are carrying around on your body and get in better shape? Sure you do. You hold the information in your conscious mind. Does this scenario sound vaguely familiar? Monday morning you wake up and start your new diet. You eat according to the plan you've chosen to follow, you get up three days that week and head to the gym and exercise, you do everything you're supposed to do for that whole week and on the following Monday you get on the scales and find that you have lost 4 pounds. You do the weight-loss happy dance around your bathroom and head off for another great week on your diet plan. But this week, somewhere around Saturday, you're at the food store and you pass the bakery and that piece of 14 layer chocolate cake starts calling your name. Or, your best friend calls and wants you to meet him at the local sports bar to watch the game and have a beer. You _KNOW_ you should not put the cake in your basket or that you should not have a beer at the bar, but you _FEEL_ like doing it. You may resist for a time, but eventually you give in to your feelings. You can _KNOW_ all day long, but in the end, if you _FEEL_ like doing something you will do it.

If what you WANT is contrary to your programming, how can you ever override your feelings long enough to get it? It all starts in your conscious mind – in choosing what information to fill your conscious mind with. In other words, choosing to think about what you want. The repetition of visualizing yourself at your ideal weight causes those paradigms that have kept you heavy to gradually change over time. Your subconscious mind has no ability to reject any idea you feed it and it has no ability to distinguish between what is real and what is imaginary. When you impress an idea on your subconscious mind over and over again, the feelings that are generated and the habits that are developed are ones that are consistent with the idea being impressed on it and you will find yourself ACTING in ways that will be consistent with achieving your desired goals.

We are all raised with a self-image—a whole collection of paradigms— that drives who we believe ourselves to be at our core. We may engage in "behavior modification" programs along the way to change a result that we don't like, but as time passes, our subconscious mind (our self-image) drives us to take actions that are consistent with whom we believe ourselves to be, thus ensuring we end up right back where we started from – or worse.

This is because we are doing nothing to change our self-image – we are just bypassing it.

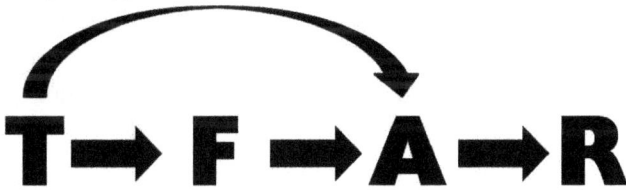

T→ F →A→R

Remember earlier we established that the thoughts we choose to consciously think about cause feelings, and the actions we take (and the subsequent results we experience) are based upon those FEELINGS, not the thoughts themselves. The only way to permanently change the behavior (and the subsequent results) is to change the self-image.

So let's get to the heart of it. There are two basic ways to alter your self-image – emotional impact and spaced repetition of ideas. Emotional impact events work fast, but you can't predict them and they are usually negative. Think about the sudden death of a loved one – the person was here just this morning and then WHAM! – he or she is gone. There is an emotional impact from an event like that – pain, sadness, grief, possibly guilt or regret. Such an event can change the way you view your world and your place in it. Spaced repetition of an idea, on the other hand, can be a slow process, but it works! It requires diligent, persistent effort, but anyone can do it and it can be a truly wonderful, positive process.

Angie is a perfect example. There was a time in her life when she was living a fairly unhealthy lifestyle. She was alone a good bit of the time and found herself unconsciously consuming large quantities of food at night. She could devour thousands of calories in a single sitting before she even realized what she was doing. As time passed and she got her life back under control, she was able to replace those bad habits with healthier ones—spending time with her family, taking an extra karate class, planning out the next day, getting extra work done—anything to keep her out of the kitchen. Now, she doesn't even consider eating outside of what is now her normal schedule for meals.

It's important to remember that we're essentially talking about changing habits here (your self-image is just a big collection of habitual patterns of thinking and acting). It's not good enough to just decide to break a bad habit. Once the bad habit is gone, what is it replaced with? Nature abhors a vacuum and releasing a bad habit leaves a void that will be filled with something. So, if you do not consciously replace a habit that it not serving you with one that will, then we can guarantee you that the void will be filled by another "bad" habit. Research has show that it takes 30-90 days to form a new habit. We'll talk more about that and give you the tools you need to replace the bad with the good later in the book, we promise!!

Embracing Fear, Doubt and Worry

It sounds pretty easy, right? All you need to do to have the body and life of your dreams is just consciously think the right thoughts and hold that vision of what you want on the screen of your mind to the exclusion of all else. Okay! Got it! No problem! Pretty simple, right? Well, there's one other piece we need to make you aware of – because once you ARE aware of what happens, you will be able to combat it. Let's say you're doing everything right – you are visualizing your perfect body, you're eating right, you're exercising, you suddenly notice your pants are a bit looser – IT'S WORKING!! Hallelujah!! And then one day WHAM!!!!! - you find yourself scared to death. Fear, doubt, worry, anxiety creep in every time you start thinking about this new life that exists in your mind and is beginning to manifest in your body. You hear a little voice inside your head saying, "You can't POSSIBLY lose all this weight – you've failed every other time - why do you think this time will be any different? And, oooooohhhhhhh wouldn't a piece of chocolate cake be AMAZING right about now? You've had a tough week, just sleep in and forget about the gym today. Who the heck do you think you are anyway – you're fat and you've always been fat and you'll always BE fat!!" Well, my friend, you have just smacked head-long into what our coach and mentor, Bob Proctor, calls THE TERROR BARRIER!!!!

First of all, CONGRATULATIONS!!! Jump up and down and CELEBRATE these feelings and know that you are closer to your goal than you have ever been before!! The terror barrier is what happens when your dream, your vision, your WHY (whatever you want to call it) begins to seep into your subconscious mind. Remember, the subconscious mind is where all the old conditioning, the paradigms, the habits and the self-image that have kept you stuck live. We affectionately call the old paradigms "Mr. X." Mr. X is very territorial and your new big dream that is seeping into your subconscious mind - let's call it "Mr. Y"- is horning in on Mr. X's space. That voice that tells you that you can't do it is Mr. X - the fear, doubt and anxiety are his weapons to get you to run back to the safety and comfort of your old paradigm and kick Mr. Y (the new idea) out of your subconscious mind.

But, if you persist and keep going and crash through the terror barrier - keep visualizing your perfect body, continue to think about it and use your burning desire for it as fuel to continue IN SPITE of the fear and the doubt - Mr. X will get weaker and weaker over time. The fear will diminish and the vision (Mr. Y) will get stronger. And then you know what happens? The "Y" idea becomes your NEW paradigm. How awesome is that!! You will end up with the self-image of a person with a lean, strong, healthy body and great nutrition and exercise habits!! What this also means is that you have to start over and build a new, even bigger vision because "Y" has now become your new "X." Do you follow me here? Remember, you're either creating or you're disintegrating – you can't stand still - you have to always be reaching for something beyond the here and now. That doesn't mean you can't be happy with where you are, but it does mean you should never be "satisfied"; you should always be striving for growth.

We spend a lot of time with clients helping them to understand one very important truth – you become what you think about. If you are thinking about what you want in life, we can assure you that you will attract it to you. However, if you are spending time thinking about what you DON'T want we can assure with just as great a level of certainty that you will keep getting more of THAT! The easiest way to explain it is to compare yourself to a magnet and realize that your thoughts and your feelings control your polarity – whether you are attracting positive to you or negative. At your most basic state you are just a large mass of energy and so is everything else – the chair you are sitting in, the keyboard you type on, the sandwich you had for lunch – all just a big mass of energy molecules moving at varying amplitudes of vibration - the more solid an object, the faster and narrower the vibratory rate.

Energy fields have a "charge" – an attractive force, and since you are essentially an energy field, YOU have positive or negative charge too. Your thoughts and feelings control that charge – the amplitude of vibration at which your body is moving. When you are feeling happy and like everything is hitting on all 8 cylinders, do you ever stop to notice that it seems like nothing can go wrong – more good just seems to come your way? You wake up feeling awesome and the kids and spouse are more cooperative and accommodating, it seems there is less traffic on the drive to work, your boss gives you a great compliment on the presentation you made the day before, and so on – it's just a great day!

The same can be said when you are having a bad day. You get out of bed, stub your toe on the bed frame, get shampoo in your eyes, burn the toast, leave the house late because Sally refused to get dressed, get stuck in a huge traffic snarl and get yelled at by your boss because you're late to work, and so on. The best way we know of to control your vibratory rate is to monitor how you are feeling. FEELING is the word we use to describe the conscious awareness of our vibratory state. Cool, huh? So if you find yourself feeling bad, do whatever you can to turn your mood around because your low vibratory rate is attracting all kinds of nastiness to you.

Stay in a Good Mood, Stay Healthy?

Let us tell you a little secret that has served us well... Did you know that viruses and bacteria and all those little germs and critters that make you sick vibrate on a very low level? If you are vibrating on a consistently high level (you are generally a happy, cheerful, upbeat, optimistic, positive person) it will be nearly impossible for you to get sick. Your authors have a lot of speaking engagements and meet and shake hands with hundreds of people, but we very rarely get sick. Deb has literally been coughed and sneezed on by people who were obviously quite ill and has never even gotten a sniffle. The opposite is true too though. We are absolutely human and definitely get in a blue funk every now and then. We recall one time that Angie had a particularly nasty bout of PMS that lasted for several days – foul mood, impatient, negative outlook, generally miserable – and a few days later she woke up with a horrible cold. The same has happened to Deb on a rare occasion. We're pretty sure the medical community would say we're nuts for such a suggestion, but since we're not doctors, who cares – it works for us and countless other people we know. Stay in a good mood and expect to stay healthy and you will!!

The more you consciously shift your destructive paradigms, the more freedom you have to make your own choices and live your own life. The subconscious mind is your central command center and each thought you allow to enter inevitably has an effect on you. Any thought you consciously choose to impress upon the subconscious mind over and over again becomes fixed in this part of your personality. When you look in the mirror do you turn away in disgust or tell yourself that you're fat? The more you think it, the easier this false belief becomes a reality. Next time, find SOMETHING about your body that you appreciate – no matter how small or insignificant it may seem - and focus on that. Be grateful for the magnificent body you've been given and know that you are getting better each and every day. Again, it goes back to belief – do you BELIEVE you can do it? Your mind is powerful and magnificent and when properly understood can bring you unlimited success. Focus all of your thoughts on what you want in life rather than what you don't want. Your results are a reflection of your self-image. By learning to apply this knowledge to your life, you will come to realize that you are in control of your own destiny and the sky is the limit.

CHAPTER TWO

Getting Your Mind Right
– Putting it all into Action

Embarking on a weight release journey can be compared to going on vacation. When most people decide to take a vacation, they sit down and make some decisions and some plans. Where do you want to go? How do you want to travel (direct, fastest route in a jet, or take your time and drive and see the countryside along the way)? What do you need to take with you? And on it goes. Well, your weight release program is no different. First of all you have your starting point – that's where you are right now – whatever your current weight, health, physical condition may be. Then you need to decide where you want to go – what's your destination? Without a clear destination, how will you ever get there. Again, think about taking a trip. You load your packed suitcases and your family or friends in the car, turn the key and get to the end of the driveway. Without a predetermined destination, which way do you turn? Often times, especially if you have been overweight and/or out of shape for a long time, it is extremely difficult to decide where you want to go. You know you need to lose weight and be healthier and more physically fit, but what does that look like? What does it FEEL like? As we have established earlier in the book, your body does not move into action based on what you know, but based upon what you FEEL. So you have to get emotionally involved in this process.

This section gives you an abundance of tools for determining your destination (your weight release goal) and then getting completely emotionally involved with that destination. We'll deal with the plan later in the book.

Tool #1: Where Are You Going?

On the following pages are some questions that will help you construct the image of your destination – your ideal weight, body, health – *your* reason for wanting to release the extra weight that is on your body. Remember, we think in pictures – it is the ONLY way we think, so the only way your mind can take your desire and move it into reality is if it has a picture to work with. These 9 questions are designed to get your dreamers turned on and worked out a little bit (most people's dream machines are rusty and creaky from disuse). Spend some focused time with them and be specific and detailed – give your subconscious mind some "meat on the bone" to chew on. If you want to release weight don't just write "I want to lose some weight." First of all, you don't "lose" weight, you *release* it (you don't want to find it again, do you?) and second, the subconscious mind needs specifics – with such a general statement, if you lose an ounce you have lost SOME weight – the universe has done its part and you're done. Instead, how much weight do you want to lose? What does your body look like when you get there? How do you feel? What kinds of things are you doing then that you aren't (or can't) do now? How does your new body perform? What are people saying to you? Are you a role model for others? How do your social interactions change? Get specific so that if someone else read what you wrote, they would see the same picture in their mind that you see in yours – the more detail, the better!

1. Why do you want to release weight?

_____

_____

_____

2. In what ways will your life be different when you have reached your ideal weight?

_____

_____

_____

_____

3. Imagine you are holding Aladdin's lamp in your hands and you are granted three wishes and that you are guaranteed to be completely successful. What do you dare to dream about your weight release if you are guaranteed success?

_____

_____

_____

_____

4. What one thing are you looking forward to most when you reach your ideal weight?

_____

_____

_____

5. What have you always wanted to do, but were afraid to try?

_____

_____

_____

_____

6. Assume for a moment that money is no object and you are at your perfect weight. What does your perfect wardrobe look like?

_____

_____

_____

_____

7. Who do you want to be – how do you want to see yourself?

_____

_____

_____

_____

_____

8. What are your talents and how are you using them? How do you WANT to use them?

_____

_____

_____

_____

9. What would make you jump out of bed every morning, excited about the day ahead?

_____

_____

_____

_____

Now that you have cranked up your "dream machine," use the feelings that you have generated to write a detailed description of as many facets of your life as you can think of once you have achieved your ideal weight and physicality.

We call this process "imagineering" and we'll go into it in great detail later in the book in the *Spirit* section because it is something that you want to incorporate into your daily life – just like taking a shower or brushing your teeth.

Here are the rules:

1. Start your vision statement with "I am so happy and grateful now that I ..." Your description should be in the present tense, as if you are living that life right now.

2. Be vivid and detailed in your narrative – to the point that a stranger could read it and have the same image in their mind that you see in yours. The more detailed you are, the clearer the image in your mind, the quicker you will see results!

3. Give absolutely NO energy to what you don't want – only consider what you DO want.

4. Remember that this is a dream, a fantasy – make sure you are writing what you really WANT, not what you think you can get – not what you think you SHOULD be happy with – it's all about what you WANT!!! Put your logic aside and have fun!

Deb Cheslow & Angie Flynn

_____

_____

_____

_____

_____

_____

_____

_____

_____

_____

_____

_____

_____

_____

_____

_____

_____

_____

_____

_____

_____

_____

_____

Read and re-read your vision statement over and over again – as often as you can. BURN the image of the life you want into your subconscious mind. As this happens, the image of what you want will take root in your subconscious and you will begin to act in ways that are consistent with your vision and following your *Release* Plan will be effortless and pleasurable. And that's when the fun REALLY begins.

However, it bears repeating, changing something as deeply ingrained in you as your self-image requires a great deal of introspection. You can't skip steps – each of the exercises is designed for a very specific reason and you have to do them all – you can't skip the parts that make you uncomfortable. In fact, the more uncomfortable the question makes you, the MORE you need to do it!! And just *thinking* about the question and answering it in your mind doesn't cut it, you **MUST** *write it down*. You see, writing causes thinking, thinking generates images, the images stir the emotions (the feelings) and those feelings drive you into action and then those actions create results. So, no short cuts! Answer all the questions, in writing; look deep inside yourself and know that if you really want to change, you will!

Tool #2: MyReleasePlan.com

The more thought energy you give to this process, the faster you will succeed. The trick is to surround yourself with like-minded people, live it, think it, breathe it and BELIEVE it! The easiest way to do this is with *MyReleasePlan.com*. Your authors are absolutely committed to your success and want to help you get phenomenal results FAST!! *MyReleasePlan.com* is a membership service that we have developed to keep your "head in the game." It is designed to expand your awareness of concepts that will continue to facilitate your self-image change. Email and video lessons with weekly exercises, live conference calls with us each month, expanded Release Plan nutrition and exercise resources, blogs, etc. *MyReleasePlan.com* will keep your vibration high and keep you focused on your goal.

Tool #3: Grab a Partner

Back in 1993 a study was conducted at Brigham Young University related to goal achievement. The study found that the probability of achieving a particular goal was associated with the statements a person made about the goal. People who said "That's a good idea" had a 10% chance. Those who said "I'll do it," had a 25% chance of reaching their goal. Those who put a date by which they planned to achieve their goal had a 40% chance of doing so. Those who developed a specific plan for reaching their goal had a 50% chance of getting there. Those who committed to someone else that they would accomplish their goal had a 60% chance of making it. But those people who committed to someone else and also committed to share their progress at regular intervals had a _95%_ chance of reaching their goal!!

The power of accountability is incredible and, as you can see, greatly increases your chances of doing what you say you are going to do. This is one reason why it is so important to have a coach or a mentor. How many times have you made a commitment to yourself, but then let yourself off the hook when the going got tough? It is next to impossible for you to see past your own logic! Does that mean you need to run to the phone and hire a your coach? Not necessarily, but it does mean that you should absolutely, positively want to be a part of our _MyReleasePlan.com_ membership service! Also, finding an "accountability partner" can be one of the most powerful things you can do if you REALLY want to reach a particular goal. We like a quote we read: "Accountability bridges the gap between intention and results!"

Finding the right accountability partner is critical. It should be someone you can trust with your dreams and someone whose opinion you value and for whom you have great respect (in other words it would hurt to let them down). In some cases it could be a best friend or a spouse (sometimes, however, those people could be the very WORST accountability partners), a business colleague, a networking associate, etc. **You** have to be willing to commit to what you wish to be held accountable for and to sharing your progress at regular intervals and **they** have to be willing to hold your feet to the fire and carry through with the consequence if need be. Your Accountability Partner must agree to request progress reports from you at an agreed upon interval of time. If left to you to provide these updates, you would likely forget all about them – this is your paradigm's way of insuring that you stay stuck right where you are.

Accountability without consequence is meaningless. Some may say, "Well, the consequence for not meeting my deadline is that I don't reach my goal," and that's true, but as human beings we are pleasure seekers and pain avoiders. It is our experience that accountability contracts that have a clearly defined consequence for non-performance work best. The consequence needs to be a source of more pain than the tasks associated with what you're being held accountable for.

Deb's Story: Here is a great example of accountability in action. Back in February my partner, Angie, was really struggling with the manuscript for this very book, Release. It is an important body of work that will help many people and we really wanted to get it finished. She had an aggressive (but doable) goal of finishing the manuscript by the end of April, but the days kept slipping away and other things kept getting in the way of the writing time. She came to me and asked me to be her accountability partner regarding the manuscript deadline. We brainstormed consequences and it quickly became obvious what that consequence needed to be. You see, Angie's happiness isn't tied to "things". We have a good life and taking away stuff or delaying getting more stuff is not much of a motivator for her. But Angie does have a burning desire and it lies in her love of karate. She was due to test for her 2nd level brown belt at our training center in Virginia in mid-May. As her instructor, I had the ability to suspend that test just by sending an email. So, the consequence of not finishing the manuscript by April 30th was the forfeit of her ability to test for her next belt in May. She came up with the consequence and her hand shook as she signed the agreement, but once she did I saw a fire in her eyes. Not only did Angie meet her deadline, but she actually turned the finished manuscript over to the internal review team 3 weeks ahead of schedule!

If you have a goal that you REALLY want to accomplish, *carefully* select an accountability partner, define and date what you are being held accountable for and devise a consequence that will cause more pain than whatever you have to do to meet your deadline. A sample Accountability Agreement is shown on the following page (and is available for download at *MyReleasePlan. com*) that will get you started. Remember the quote we used earlier – "Accountability bridges the gap between intention and results." An accountability agreement moves intention from a mere wish to a near certainty. GO FOR IT!!

ACCOUNTABILITY AGREEMENT

THIS AGREEMENT is entered into by and between _____
("Participant") and _____ ("Accountability Partner") this
_____ day of _____, 20_____. In consideration of the
mutual promises made in this agreement, the parties agree as follows:

1. Participant pledges and agrees to perform the action detailed below
   by the date specified and to be accountable to the Accountability
   Partner for progress reports at _____
   intervals.

   Action Step   **Due Date**
   _____   _____

2. Accountability Partner agrees to hold Participant accountable for
   the performance of the action listed above by the specified date and
   to request progress reports from Participant at the interval detailed
   above.

3. Failure of Participant to comply with request for progress reports by
   Accountability Partner in a timely manner constitutes a breach of
   this Agreement; however, failure to meet incremental action plans
   that may be agreed upon between progress report updates does not
   constitute a breach of the Agreement, per se.

4. Both Participant and Accountability Partner acknowledge that
   accountability without consequence is meaningless and agree to the
   following consequence for non-performance. Accountability Partner
   accepts the responsibility for enforcing the consequence.

Consequence for Non-Performance
_____
_____
_____

My signature indicates my understanding and acceptance of this
Agreement.

Participant   **Accountability Partner**

_____   _____
Printed Name   Printed Name

_____   _____
Signature   Signature

_____   _____
Date   Date

Tool #4: Using a Daily Commitment Sheet

Almost 100 years ago a management consultant named Ivy Lee was doing some work with Charles Schwab, the head of Bethlehem Steel at the time. Schwab was lamenting that his biggest obstacle to true, runaway success in the steel business was in the effectiveness of his management team – they just didn't do a very good job of utilizing their time. Lee told Schwab that in 20 minutes he could show him a technique that would multiply the effectiveness and productivity of himself and his entire team. Schwab asked him how much it would cost and Lee said that was up to him - to try it for a few weeks and then to send him a check for whatever he thought it was worth. Schwab gave Lee the go-ahead to spend 20 minutes with each member of his team to introduce his system. A few weeks later Schwab sent Lee a check for $25,000 (that's easily equivalent to ~$250,000 today) as compensation for the tool he had provided them with.

Here is Lee's system as it was given to the executives at Bethlehem Steel in the 1920's: Each evening before leaving your office take a blank Commitment form and write down, in order of priority, the top 6 things you will do the following day that will help you move toward your goal. They should be achievable during the following day. Clear your desk of all extraneous papers except for your Daily Commitment Sheet and leave the office.

The next morning when you come to the office take your list and start with #1 on the list. Give no thought to #2, just give your full focus and attention to #1. When #1 is complete, move to #2 on the list. Give no thought to #1 and do not anticipate #3, just focus on #2 until it is complete. Then move to #3… Work through the list in this manner until your list is complete. Before you leave the office at the end of the day, complete a commitment sheet for the next day.

Now, obviously Lee's system was designed for application in a workplace setting, but most of us do not have the option of turning our pursuit of a lean, strong, healthy body into our full time job. So how do you make this tool work for you when there are so many other things you HAVE to do on a daily basis? How do you apply Lee's system in that case? Well, here's the answer: It is important to understand that your Daily Commitment Sheet is NOT a day-planner – it is not your schedule. It is to be completed with the constraints of the next day's schedule in mind. Let's look at an example. Let's assume that, your day planner for tomorrow looks something like this:

7:00   Take child to the bus stop
9:30   Staff Meeting
11:00   Sales Presentation
12:30   Lunch with Bill Smith (XYZ Corp)
2:00   Admin Time in Office
4:00   Sales Presentation
5:30   Pick up child from After-School Care
7:00   Family Dinner

On the surface, there doesn't seem to be a lot of free time for "goal achieving" activities, does there? But remember, we're not talking about leaping from the starting point to the manifestation of your perfect body in one day – not at all!! This is about choosing 6 things – no matter how small – that will advance you a fraction of a baby step toward your ultimate goal. Now, that said, you don't put items on the list that you do habitually – you wouldn't put "Brush teeth" on your commitment sheet, because that's a habit and you would do it anyway. So, given the schedule constraints for the day, the items that go on the Daily Commitment Sheet might be:

1. Go to the gym – Cardio workout
2. Plan menu for next week
3. Shop for free day food (we'll explain this later – you're going to LOVE it!!)
4. Make a double batch of dinner and freeze it for a busy night
5. Read *MyReleasePlan.com* article on modified abdominal exercises
6. Research new plan-friendly lunch ideas on internet

None of these items are incredibly time consuming, but they are still prioritized. You can go to the gym as soon as you wake up. Plan your menu for the next week after your shower. Shop for free day food on your way to pick up the kids from after school care. You're going to make dinner anyhow, so making an extra batch doesn't take any more time at all. And finally, you can read the article and conduct the internet research after the kids go to bed. You can see that even though none of these activities are earth shattering on their face, each is an action oriented task that moves you a little closer to your goal. When you are prioritizing your tasks for the next day, push yourself even harder and choose the task that makes you most uncomfortable and make that the #1 thing you will do! Make a habit of attacking the thing that you least want to do first – it will not only get it out of the way up front (helping to keep your vibration high), but it will also kill that tendency to procrastinate!!

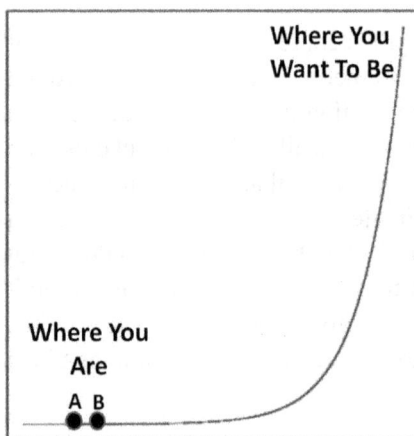

We talk a lot about focusing on the ultimate goal and you absolutely should be as often as possible throughout the day. But when you are completing your Daily Commitment Sheet, your 6 commitments should be absolutely logical and planned – you can see the next step and you know what you need to do to complete it. If you look at your goal on a graph, it looks something like the figure on the left.

Where You Want To Be

Where You Are

A B

You have no idea how you are going to get from where you are right now to where you want to ultimately be – it is exponential growth, it is illogical, but look at points A and B – they're right beside each other – B is only very slightly higher than A – you can logically SEE and PLAN how to move from point A to point B. THAT'S what we're talking about with your daily commitments – planned, achievable, action oriented tasks that move you along the curve from day to day. However, it is CRITICAL that you always have your ultimate vision – your GOAL - in mind. Without it, you will "logic yourself to death." You will work on these 6 tasks each day that are planned and very linear, but you will never follow the curve upwards toward your goal. You'll just keep plodding along, day after day, on what seems like a straight line, but in fact, since nothing can stand still - you are either creating or disintegrating - if you are not following the curve up to your goal, you are actually going backwards – disintegrating. To illustrate the point graphically, your progress actually looks like this:

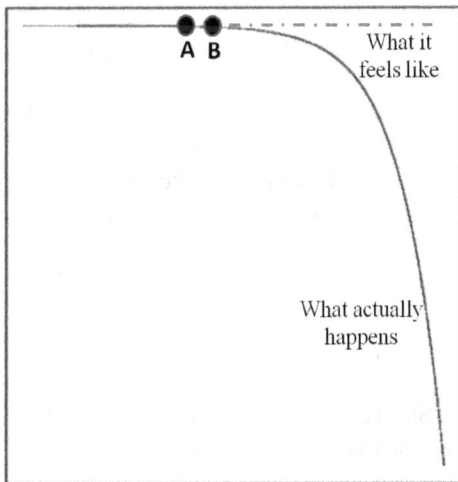

You have to keep upping the ante, so to speak, and the only way to make sure that you are tackling the tasks that will move you along that upward curve to your goal is to constantly have that vision in your mind and keep asking yourself, "Will this action (this task or commitment) take me closer to my goal?" If the answer is "Yes," then great - do it; however, if the answer is "No" pick another task for your Daily Commitment Sheet.

One last point about the items you choose for your Daily Commitment Sheet. We've mentioned that the tasks need to be achievable within the day. PLEASE do not use your Daily Commitment Sheet as a "stick!" In other words, don't get wrapped up in the idea that you need to put items on your list to FORCE yourself to do them. Force negates everything and if you are putting things on your list that would be better served by waiting for a day when you have a large block of time to devote to them, please wait! For example, if your goal was to participate in a marathon 6 months from now and your day planner for tomorrow looked like the one on page 59, you wouldn't want to list

"Run half marathon" as one of your 6 items – there's just not enough time in the day to accomplish it – unless you want to run in the dark, but you might list "Run 2 miles" on your list – that could easily be done in 30 minutes or less. Save your half marathon for the weekend when your schedule is less cramped. It is critically important that your list be achievable. We are not suggesting you procrastinate; however, we are saying do not use your commitment sheet as a means of forcing square pegs into round holes.

Let's discuss for a moment the habits that using this tool will foster.

1. Prioritization: Knowing not only what you need to do, but also what is most important is an essential goal achieving quality.

2. Productivity and Effectiveness: Ending each day by completing your Daily Commitment Sheet allows your subconscious mind to see what's coming for the next day and, at the same time be focused on your goal. Your subconscious mind will literally work on the various tasks all night long while you sleep. You will find that you will wake up with intuitive bursts that will help you move toward your goal – and get your list accomplished!

3. Success: When you have the experience of having all 6 items on your Daily Commitment Sheet checked off day after day, you build a success mindset (rather than working from that ponderous "To Do" list that all of us have that never seems to get any shorter and makes you feel like you're spinning your wheels). Regardless of what else happened that day, you completed the 6 most important things that will move you toward your goal – the day was a success. Success breeds success. One day will build on the next and before you know it you will find that your goal has manifested!

4. Keeping Commitments: Most people fall into one of two camps when it comes to making and keeping their commitments. They are either not very good at keeping commitments to anyone OR they are good at keeping the commitments they make to other people, but they are not very good at keeping the commitments they make to themselves. By completing your Daily Commitment Sheet and checking off each item every day, you are building the habit of

making and KEEPING commitments to yourself (and that's what the day-to-day nit-noids of the *Release* Plan are all about – making and keeping commitments to yourself to do the work)!! This is so huge!! Just imagine what your life would be if every time you said "I should…" you actually DID!!

In summary, here's how to use your Daily Commitment Sheet (download a Template and instructions at *MyReleasePlan.com*):

- Before going to bed each day make a prioritized list of the 6 things you need to do the following day to move toward your goal within the constraints of your schedule;
- The next day, as pockets of time are available begin working on task #1 with your full focus until it is complete;
- Then move on to task #2 – no attention to #1, no anticipation of #3;
- Proceed through your list until all 6 items are complete;
- Congratulate yourself on a job well done; and
- Make a list for the next day.

We use the Daily Commitment Sheet in our work life and it has made a tremendous difference in our effectiveness and productivity. We encourage you to apply this concept to other areas of your life. You see, you can apply the knowledge that you have just received about your mind to any area of your life where you would like to improve your results – whether it's your weight, your relationships, your income, your spirituality – ANYTHING!! It all works together.

MY DAILY COMMITMENTS

I, _____, commit to complete the following six tasks that will move me closer to my goals by the end of today, _____, 20_____.

Number One	☐ Complete

Number Two	☐ Complete

Number Three	☐ Complete

Number Four	☐ Complete

Number Five	☐ Complete

Number Six	☐ Complete

"Every action we take, everything we do is either a victory or defeat in the struggle to become what we want to be."

-Ninon de L'Enclos

Your signature is a symbol of the commitment you have made to yourself for today. In learning to keep our commitments, not only to others, but also to ourselves, we find the journey to the attainment of our goals is a much smoother, straighter line.

_____
Signature

Courtesy of Deb Cheslow Consulting
www.DebCheslow.com (386)308-2155
©2012 Deb Cheslow Consulting

Tool #5: When Life Gets in the Way – Put it in a Box

We know that no matter how much you might like for life to be smooth sailing, it just doesn't play out that way 24/7. We hear from clients all the time who want to know how to handle it when life throws them a curveball. The conversation starts something like this: "I understand that I have to keep my vibration high and I have to focus on what I want and I have to hold the image of my ideal body on the screen of my mind with my will and all that. I GET it, but how do I DO it when everyday life gets in the way and my bank account is down to $10 and there are 10 days left until payday and my daughter just broke curfew for the third time this week and my husband forgot to take out the garbage and I just feel like the whole world is falling down around me?"

We LOVE this question because this is something we have to contend with every day in our own lives and the answer literally transformed our lives! In our business, we work with people, groups and entire companies to help them develop the mindset to create the results that they want. In order to do that, we have to be 100% focused on THEM in our sessions. We have to actively listen and allow intuition to enable us to guide them on their journey. We cannot allow ourselves to be thinking about our daughter's boyfriend issues or our son's behavior marks in school, or the presidential election or WHATEVER "junk" might be going on in our personal lives. If we are absorbed with OUR junk, how can we possibly help someone else move past theirs?

So, we have developed the habit of putting all our personal "junk" in a container before we go into a session. We actually sit back and relax and picture taking all our issues and putting them in a container (and some days we have to really STUFF that puppy full), put the lid on and then place it on an imaginary shelf. Then, with our minds clear, we are able to focus on whatever lies ahead – whether that be working with a client, spending quality time with our family – whatever. We have permission to go back and pop the lid off the box and reengage all our junk at a later time if we choose to.

Deb Cheslow & Angie Flynn

What we have discovered is that when we employ this technique we are much calmer, better focused, more effective individuals. And, best of all, when we do go back and open up the container we often find that the problems that seemed so overwhelming previously were actually not such a big deal after all. Remember, what you think about comes about, so if you keep thinking about your problems, you will get more problems! But, if you think about what you want and focus on the task at hand, you place yourself in a creative position and a positive vibration – and then, dear reader, you find solutions!

When life gets crazy and overwhelming we encourage you to just put it all in a box. Visualize yourself taking whatever is bothering you and physically stuffing it into a box. Pop the lid on, put it on a shelf and focus on the task at hand. You can always come back to your troubles later if you really want to.

CHAPTER THREE

Watch out for the Crabs

We came across a fantastic essay by Susan Raines-Bridges called "The Miracle of the Crab Pot" that really speaks to the power of paradigms as they relate to you and those who are closest to you. It uses the metaphor of the way crabs behave when they are caught at sea by crab fishermen. When these fisherman head out to sea, they cast out big nets and bring in great quantities of crabs onto the fishing boat where they are placed in great big holding pots. The instinct of most of the crabs is to make a pile in the center of the pot and build a pyramid to the top of the pot. The crabs will wrestle very aggressively to get to the top of the heap, often maiming or killing other crabs along the way, only to find that when they get to the top of the pile they are no closer to freedom than they were at the bottom because they are still too far away from the edge to escape. Occasionally, a crab with a different instinct will start climbing up the side of the pot – which is, of course, the only way to freedom. The pots, over time, get dings and nicks in the sides so the crab is able to get a foothold and carefully scale the side of the pot. When one of the crabs in the heap notices the crab going up the sides, s/he will leave the pile and come over to the side and yank the wayward crab off the wall, back to the bottom of the pot where s/he "belongs."

Have you ever noticed that people tend to behave in very similar ways? Think about it for a moment... Have you ever tried to climb out of your "pot" – that place where you are comfortable and where everyone who knows you best is comfortable with you being? For example, you're reading this book, which means that somewhere along the way you decided that the image reflected back at you in the mirror is not one you are pleased with. Does this scenario sound vaguely familiar? As your weight starts to go down family and friends express their delight at your resolve and offer their support and best wishes for your success. If you manage to fight your own conditioning long enough for your actions to really start being noticeable, all of a sudden these same relatives and friends subtly begin sabotaging your efforts. Mom has your favorite forbidden foods available when you come for a visit, a best friend chooses a place for lunch where there is nothing plan-friendly on the menu, your spouse or significant other ties up your time so you have difficulty fitting in time at the gym. If you are able to withstand the pressure and persist with your plan, the subtly of the sabotage becomes progressively more aggressive – negative comments about looking gaunt or ill, belittling your efforts by bringing up past failures, pushing you to eat foods you shouldn't or risk "hurting their feelings." Eventually, the pressure becomes an all out assault – relationships can even be severed or sorely damaged because of your unwillingness to bend to familial or social pressure.

It's much like the crabs in the above mentioned crab pot. Those closest to you – who say they want the very best for you - see you trying to "get out of the pot" – trying to better yourself in some way, and they do their damnedest to pull you right off the wall, back into your "pot" – where they are comfortable with you – where you (in their mind) belong!

You persist, braving their displeasure, ignoring their comments, and they pull out all the stops. They tell you and anyone else who will listen that there is something wrong with you – in the case of a prolonged weight control program, perhaps they insinuate that you have an eating disorder or some other physical or emotional problem.

You try to share what you are learning with them, but, locked on their own perspective, their brains refuse to accept any part of the knowledge you are gaining. They absolutely, passionately refuse to acknowledge how you are changing. To them, your 'assigned' role is cast in stone.

At some point you are forced to make a choice – abandon your quest for change and once again take your place in the "pot"; or, you can finally get to the uppermost point in your life (the top of the crab pot) and decide to fall outside the pot.

So, to continue the crabbing analogy, what happens when the rare crab makes it to the top of the pot and pulls himself over the edge and lands on the ship's deck? Does the crab fisherman pick him up and throw him back in the pot? No. In reality the exact opposite happens. The fisherman picks up the crab and throws him back into the ocean, setting him free. The fisherman knows that there is something special in that crab – a survival instinct that is stronger than normal. Such crabs will surely mate and pass this instinct on to their progeny, ensuring the survival of the species for generations of crab fishermen to come!

So, what happens to the person who perseveres and finally makes their way to the top of their personal 'crab pot' and pulls himself over the edge and falls to the deck? Well, that's where the magic happens – that's when you are free to create whatever big, beautiful life YOU choose. That's when you discover your own power.

Isn't that great?? Sadly, however, those who profess to love us the most and want the very best for us will be our most crafty and devious saboteurs – not because they are bad, conniving people, but because they also have paradigms and you have a particular place in those paradigms, and because they are not armed with the awareness that you now have, they act out of habit and instinct and will do whatever they can to derail your efforts.

Commit to surrounding yourself with positive people who support you in your commitment to reach your goals. We are not telling you to abandon your current friends and family, but it is critical that you recognize what may happen as you begin to make big changes in your life. In this age of the internet, you are only a couple of clicks away from positive inspiration at *MyReleasePlan. com*. If you have a "crab" in your life trying to "pull you off the wall," grab the lifeline that someone else is holding out for you.

Final Words

We have spent a lot of time in this first section of the book explaining how your mind works and why you have to develop a basic understanding of it before you can make big, quantum leap-type changes in any area of your life. You see, any big change has to start on the inside. We spend so much of our lives living from the outside in, but once we start living from the inside out, HUGE things can happen for us!

But, we'll say it again (and again and again), you can't pick and choose the parts of this book that you want to do and leave the rest behind. The more uncomfortable a question or an exercise makes you, the MORE you need to tackle it with gusto because that's where one of those nasty paradigms that is trying to keep you stuck lives. You are far too capable and intelligent to be the obstacle standing in your own way!!

NOW, let's apply what we have learned so far and get into the nuts and bolts of the *Release* Plan. Are you ready?

Body

"Each of us are our own greatest inhibitor. And, at the end of the day, if you just get out of your own way and let things come to you, it's amazing what will come to you."
–Laird Hamilton

Deb Cheslow & Angie Flynn

CHAPTER FOUR

Diets Don't Work!

How many times have you heard it - DIETS don't work – they just don't. They never have and they never will. Diets are about short term behavior that reduces calories and essentially makes your body think it's starving! It's like holding your breath underwater – eventually you have to take a breath and when you do you're sucking in all the air you possibly can. The same thing happens with food when you're on a diet. You go along just great for a while – maybe even a long while, but then your conditioning (your paradigm) catches you in a moment of weakness and you give in and you eat something you're not supposed to – or worse, you *binge* on lots of somethings! Then comes the self-reproach – the beating yourself up because you were weak – and your self-esteem takes a nosedive. The fact is that we are designed by evolution to fail on diets – period! (we'll talk about that later). There are tens of thousands of diet plans to choose from – Angie just typed "diet books" into Amazon.com's search engine and 63,582 results were returned! According to the Federal Trade Commission, 95% of people who start a weight-loss diet each year will regain all the weight they lose (or more) within one year. That's a very sad statistic, but one that bears out over and over again.

As we designed the *Release* Plan, we wanted to offer people not just another "diet" – not a program that they endure for a period of time and then abandon – but a *lifestyle* that is energizing and pleasurable and that offers exceptional results and adapts with the person's changing body, so plateaus become a thing of the past! Deb has been eating and exercising this way for over a decade with tremendous results. Angie followed the same program for over 2 years before she and Deb developed *Release* and has seen similarly dramatic results. The key is that both of us went into our programs with the mindset that this was a new lifestyle, not just another diet.

There are several things to keep in mind as you move through the Body section. We are going to introduce concepts, theories, and tools that may be brand new to you and there may be moments when you feel a bit confused and overwhelmed. Don't worry! Out of confusion comes order and all the details will be crystal clear in the end. Plus, with *MyReleasePlan.com* we'll be there with you every day to hold your hand, offer support, and answer your questions, helping you make it happen in the real world! So, our recommendation is to read this section the first time straight through so you are familiar with the basic concepts. As we said, there is a lot of new information in here and some of it is intertwined throughout multiple sections. It is impossible to introduce everything at once, so some confusion is normal. Once you've read through once, go back and re-read it – each time you do this, the plan will become exponentially clearer.

CHAPTER FIVE

How Did I Get Here?

In order to make any type of permanent change, it is critical that you examine your habitual patterns of behavior that are keeping you from achieving the results you want and then take measures to change them.

Angie: My top three habits that were sabotaging me from achieving my ideal weight day after day were:

1. *I skipped meals.*
2. *My portion sizes were too big and I ate too fast.*
3. *I wasn't drinking nearly enough water.*

Deb: I had three very obvious patterns that were keeping me from reaching my weight goals:

1. *Nonstop "grazing" on junk foods.*
2. *I ate ice cream EVERY night before bed (and had for DECADES – ever since I was a small child).*
3. *Not drinking enough water.*

Until we changed those habitual patterns, we were never going to experience the results we wanted to see on our bodies no matter how hard we worked out, because we were subtly sabotaging our efforts every single day. Our bodies didn't have what they needed in order to transform in the way we wanted them to.

Before we get into the *Release* Plan specifics, we need YOU to get real with YOU, because nothing else in this book is going to help you make a LASTING change until you do.

Sit down and relax and really think about how you go through your day. What are the things that you are doing habitually (without conscious thought) that are holding you back from achieving your weight release goals? Do you head to the cafeteria vending machines for coffee and a candy bar each morning? Do you find yourself sitting in the Starbucks drive-thru line every morning ordering a scone and a latte? Do you drink enough water throughout the day? Do you constantly put off exercise until tomorrow? Do you mindlessly munch while watching television?

Write down the 3 most prevalent habits that are holding you back.

1.

_____

_____

_____

2.

_____

_____

_____

3.

_____

_____

_____

The biggest part of getting what you want in life lies in knowing what you have to give up in order to achieve it. Now, we don't mean this from a "lack and limitation" perspective, but rather from the perspective of giving up something of a lower nature to gain something of a higher nature. So now that you have identified what's holding you back, know that those are the things you need to give up.

Here we come to another pesky little detail regarding the way the universe works – Nature abhors a vacuum. If you give up something, it leaves a vacuum – a hole – and the natural order of things is to fill the vacuum (hole) as quickly as possible. As human beings, this basic truth holds again and again – if you don't consciously replace a negative habit with a positive habit, it will be replaced with a new negative habit, subconsciously. So, now that you have identified the habits that are holding you back, you need to flip each one on its ear and turn it into a positive. For example, when Angie did this exercise and listed her 3 most prevalent negative habit patterns, her new positive habits looked like this:

1. I set a timer to indicate when I need to eat and I have my meals planned ahead of time.
2. I measure my portions and put my fork down between bites of food.
3. Every time I am eating, I must drink a 16 oz. glass of water before I finish my meal.

Now, in the space provided, turn each of your negative habits into positives:

1.

_____

_____

_____

2.

_____

_____

_____

3.

_____

_____

_____

Deb Cheslow & Angie Flynn

Awesome! Now, let's talk about the science of changing a habit for a moment. Research has shown us that it takes at least 30 days to begin to form a new habit. In fact, one of these research studies is an incredible illustration of the physiological connection between time and "habits." Back in the early days of the space program, NASA designed an experiment to determine the physiological and psychological effects of the spatial disorientation the astronauts would experience in the weightless environment of space. NASA needed to know if this environment would have some unexpected negative consequences that would endanger the astronauts or their mission. Would they black out and be unable to function? Would they experience some psychotic event that would leave them incapacitated? NASA scientists outfitted the astronauts with pairs of convex goggles which flipped everything in their field of vision 180 degrees. In other words, their world was literally turned upside down. The astronauts had to wear the goggles 24 hours a day, 7 days per week—even when they were asleep.

Although they experienced physical symptoms of anxiety and stress initially – elevated blood pressure, respiration and other vital signs, they gradually adapted to their new "realities." On the 26th day of the experiment, something amazing happened for one of the astronauts. His world turned right-side up again even though he continued to wear the goggles 24 hours a day. Between days 26-30, the same thing happened for each of the remaining astronauts. What the scientists discovered is that after 26-30 days of this continuous stream of new input the astronauts' brains actually created neural pathways that "rewired" their brains to see their worlds normally again.

Then NASA repeated the experiment with a slight change. This time the astronauts took the goggles off for a short period of time partway through the experiment. When they put the goggles back on and left them on until the 30th day, their worlds were still upside down. What the scientists discovered from these experiments is that the brain requires approximately 30 uninterrupted days for new neural connections to form – for new *habits* to form.

What this means for you in the context of your *Release* Plan is that for the first 30 days you are really going to have to consciously think about these new habits and remind yourself about them over and over again. Maybe you put post-it notes around your house to remind you to exercise or to grab a glass of water; or put a sign on your refrigerator and pantry doors to snap you out of habitual snacking. You must put systems in place to ensure you follow the new behavior you have chosen. Otherwise, *without thinking* you will revert to the old behavior! For example, Deb fills a large container with water each morning and she won't go to bed that night until the container is empty. Changing habitual actions is a fantastic place to use an accountability partner (as we discussed in the first section of this book)!

After 30 days of conscious, intentional, deliberate thought and effort it gets easier and easier and by 90 days it is very much a part of you – a new habit; only this time it's one that is serving you and moving you toward your goals. Then you can start the whole process over to change additional bad habits!

Deb Cheslow & Angie Flynn

CHAPTER SIX
Your Magnificent Body

As we've mentioned before, nothing stands still – we are in a constant state of motion – either creating or disintegrating. Your body is the perfect example of this – it is comprised of some 75 TRILLION cells, which are in a continual state of re-creation. Research shows that not one of those trillions of cells that is in your body today will be there in one year – it's like you get a completely new body every year. So, tell us, are you going to be a better version of you this time next year or a worse version? The choice is yours, but sadly, the odds are against you. The typical western (American) diet is woefully deficient in water, essential fats, protein, vitamins and minerals. Our bodies are incredible machines – new cells will continue to be created as old ones disintegrate, but without the proper building blocks they will be worse versions of cells than their predecessors. The "new you" that results from the average American diet is a worse version than the previous version. Over time this disintegrative reproduction results in (at best) low energy, aches, pains, lethargy and depression, and at worst, diseases such as diabetes and cancer.

So, are you regenerating into a better, stronger, healthier you (creating) or a worse, weaker, sicker version of yourself (disintegrating)? Think about it, if your body is in a continual state of re-creation and you are sitting on the sofa watching TV or playing video games and eating supersized fast food meals, potato chips and candy all day, do you think your body is going to be running at peak efficiency or regenerating into a healthier version of you than you were yesterday? Of course not. However, if you are exercising several times per week and eating a diet of REAL food – meats, fruits, vegetables, whole grains, eggs, and dairy products – can you see that you have a fighting chance of being a better version of yourself today than you were yesterday?

Let's get into it then. What and, as importantly, HOW do you eat?

The purpose of food, at its most basic level, is to fuel your body in a way that allows you to function at an efficient level. Of course, your societal conditioning has morphed the image of food into a comfort/pleasure source and we do not argue this point – WE LOVE FOOD!!! We want the food we eat to taste great, to hit all those comfort and pleasure centers of our brain, but also fuel our bodies in the most effective and efficient way possible. We want to choose the highest quality fuel for our body's engine.

If you start researching nutrition, it's easy to get really confused really fast. It seems that there is very little consensus among experts on what the optimal nutritional plan for human beings consists of. Some say fat is the enemy; others vilify carbohydrates; others tout the virtues of a vegetarian diet; still others say you have to combine foods to get benefits; and on and on it goes. There are, no doubt, as many "right" answers as there are "experts" on the subject. Now, while we're not necessarily "experts" in nutrition – you'll not find any certificates or diplomas on our walls – we do have a wealth of knowledge and we have developed a program that WORKS. And in the end, isn't that what matters?

Food and Your Body

In this section we're going to give you a very basic overview of how the food you are eating functions in your body. At its most basic level, the food you eat is used to fuel your body. It's like putting gas in a car – without gas the engine won't run. Every bite of food that enters your mouth, whether it is a kidney bean or a jelly bean, is broken down into one of three major (macro) nutrients: protein, carbohydrate or fat. Although each of these macronutrients provides energy for your body in one way or another, they also have many other functions (don't worry, we're not even going to attempt to go into them all here).

Protein (found in meat, poultry, fish, eggs, legumes, milk and milk products, vegetables and grains) is used by the body to build and repair your body's cells, in various enzymatic reactions, and in the production of hormones and antibodies.

Carbohydrates (found in breads, cereals, grains, pasta, rice, fruits, vegetables, milk and sugars) provide specific fuel for your brain, your nervous system and your red blood cells. Carbohydrates make it possible for the building blocks of proteins and amino acids to enter the cells to do their job by triggering the release of insulin.

Fats (found in meats, poultry, fish, milk and milk products, nuts and seeds, oils, butter, margarine, salad dressing, and most desserts) deliver other fat-soluble nutrients (vitamins), comprise parts of cell membranes and the membranes around nerve bundles, and assist in the production of hormones and bile (for fat digestion). Fats are not your enemy! Saturated fats and those nasty trans-fats (see box below) are the enemy. Unsaturated fats are actually GOOD for your body in reasonable amounts. How do you know the difference between a saturated fat and an unsaturated fat? The *general* rule is that if the fat is solid at room temperature (lard, butter, shortening) it needs to be avoided. Good fats, like safflower oil, extra-virgin olive oil and sesame oil are unsaturated – they are liquid at room temperature. Now, remember, we said *REASONABLE* amounts, so just because a fat is unsaturated doesn't mean you can eat a ton of it! Plus, if you incorporate fish in your diet a couple of times per week – especially fish like salmon, fresh tuna and halibut – you're likely getting plenty of these essential fatty acids in your nutrition plan already!

The Buzz on Trans Fats

We hear a lot about trans fats and that we should stay away from them. Why is that? Well, trans fats (named *trans* because of the stereochemistry of the functional groups in the fat molecule – we KNEW that semester of organic chemistry would come in handy some day) are created in a laboratory – they do not occur in nature. Like most things that are detrimental, when you boil it all down you find that money is at its root cause. Trans fats are no different. In a nutshell, saturated fats (fats that are solid at room temperature), like butter or lard, are the best

---

types of fat to use in baking – they yield the best end product in terms of taste and texture, but they are significantly more expensive than unsaturated fats (liquid at room temperature), like vegetable oil. Some genius in the food industry decided to head into a laboratory and start tinkering with the molecular structure of unsaturated fat (oil) and discovered a way to make it solid at room temperature – voila, the partially hydrogenated (or trans) fat was born. The result was that the food industry could produce "higher quality" baked goods at a significantly lower cost. Of course, there are always unintended consequences. Trans fats really confuse our bodies (probably because they are not natural). Our bodies treat trans fats like saturated fats and they raise LDL (bad) cholesterol levels. But trans fats have a bonus bad effect of lowering HDL (good) cholesterol levels – making it horrendously bad for you!

You need all three macronutrients – proteins, carbohydrates and fats - in your diet in order for your body to function properly and that's exactly what the *Release* Plan prescribes. The *Release* Plan is a lower-fat (not no-fat), moderate carbohydrate and moderate protein nutrition plan. The composition of *Release* Plan meals averages ~ 40% protein, 40% carbohydrate and 20% fat.

CHAPTER SEVEN

EATING: How, What, When, Why?

The *Release* Plan advocates eating 6 smaller meals per day (rather than the traditional 3 meals), each containing approximately equal portions of protein and carbohydrate (high quality, complex carbohydrates) and a vegetable (in at least at two of your daily meals), at regularly spaced intervals of 2-3 hours. Your body is an amazingly intelligent machine and it will tell you what it needs if only you will LISTEN to it! Think about it, when do you find yourself hungry? For us it's shortly after waking up, then somewhere around 10:00 in the morning, again around 12:30-1:00pm, then the dreaded afternoon slump around 3:00pm, then again around 6:00pm, and we get a little peckish before bed around 9:00pm. Our body tells us that it is in need of additional fuel every 2-3 waking hours – it just does.

We would be very interested in knowing WHO decreed it part of the human condition that *thou shalt eat 3 meals per day*. Seriously, it's just another paradigm – a habitual pattern that someone back in the gene pool started following and they taught it to their children, and they taught it to *their* children and so on and so on until our parents taught it to US. You believe it to be correct because it's what you've always done, but when really examined, does it make the most sense? We don't think so – not at all! Let's start listening to our bodies and feeding them when they require fuel (as communicated through that uncomfortable grumbling in our belly when we get hungry). Since our bodies tend to show signs of needing fuel 6 times per day anyhow, darn it, let's buck the system and eat 6 times per day, okay? We need to throw in a caveat here… If you have been skipping meals for a long period of time, your body may have very well adjusted to eating only once or twice per day and you may not feel hungry throughout the day. We urge you to consider the "sense" in eating this way. If you are reading this book, it's likely that YOUR approach has not gotten you where you desire to be. Einstein defined insanity as doing the same thing over and over expecting a different result. Why not shake things up a bit and try something that makes sense AND WORKS!!

Fun Fact

The phrase "3 square meals per day" originated back in the days of wooden sailing vessels. The crew was served their meals on square, wooden plates (that would not break if they fell off the tables when the seas were rough). The goal was to make sure the crew received several hot, edible meals per day, but that was often impossible due to poor weather conditions or lack of provisions. So if the crew received "3 squares a day" they considered themselves to be doing very well.

Remember, this is a LIFESTYLE, not just another "diet." Do you hear what we're saying here? You have to eat more often in order to release weight! Does that excite you? It should!

Of course, eating twice as many times as we are used to per day means we need to take a look at how MUCH we are eating at each of those meals. Unfortunately, 97% of the population of the Western world needs some serious re-education on portion sizes. Super-sized fast food meals and the entrée portions that are served at most restaurants are NOT single servings. We dare say we could feed our family of 4 from one entrée at some of these eateries! Eating 6 meals in those amounts won't EVER get you where you want to go, so you will need to correct your portion distortion. And NO, we are not going to tell you that you need to run out and buy a food scale and a bunch of special gadgets to make sure you're eating the right amount of food – all you need is one hand. A proper serving size of protein is a piece that is roughly the size of the palm of your hand (½" – ¾" thick) . A proper serving of carbohydrate is roughly the size of your clenched fist. A serving of hard cheese or peanut butter is roughly the size of your thumb. The cool thing about measuring food portions this way is that it is self adjusting – if you are a 5'0" tall woman, you will require smaller portions than a 6'5" tall man – but guess what, your hand is going to be one heck of a lot smaller than his too, so the measurements hold.

Measuring this way also means you don't really have to worry about calories. If you are eating foods that are on the *Endorsed Foods* list (which is by no means all-inclusive) in the proper portion sizes at the appropriate times during the day, the number of calories you are eating will take care of itself. This is incredibly freeing (and maybe just a little bit disconcerting) for people who have made it their business to know the calorie content of every food in their pantry. Think about how much thought energy you can devote to other areas of your life when you don't have to calculate calories every day!! Now, what you do need to watch is protein and carbohydrate content – only because they need to be roughly equal at each meal. We suggest you shoot for 20 grams of protein and 20 grams of carbohydrate (Amount of Total Carb minus Fiber) at each of your 6 meals. Don't worry about getting obsessive-compulsive about it – just use the 20/20 Rule as a guideline.

Why the Protein/Carbohydrate Balance?

There is a physiological reason for the protein/carb balance. In a nutshell, amino acids (the building blocks of protein) can only enter your cells to help regenerate and rebuild them when insulin is released. The carbohydrates you eat trigger the release of insulin. Quality carbohydrates and protein work together to ensure proper cellular function – that's why you need BOTH at every meal. And this is also why diets that promote severe restriction of carbohydrates are not good for your body.

What Can I Eat?
RELEASE Plan Endorsed Foods
Proteins

Poultry
- Skinless chicken breast
- Skinless turkey breast

Fish
- Tilapia
- Cod
- Haddock
- Tuna, canned, water packed and fresh
- Salmon canned, water packed and fresh
- Shellfish (crab, shrimp, lobster, clams, scallops)

Beef
- Lean ground beef (< 10% fat)
- Buffalo
- Round steak
- Sirloin steak

Lean ham
Eggs (preferably organic), egg whites and egg substitutes (like Egg Beaters)
Skim milk (preferably organic)
Low-fat cheeses
Nonfat Greek yogurt
Low-fat or fat-free cottage cheese
Nuts (cashews, almonds,macadamia, peanut)

Carbohydrates

Potatoes (red, white, yellow, blue, sweet)
Squash (spaghetti squash, acorn squash, pumpkin)
Corn
Brown rice (cooked without oil or butter)
Whole grain pasta
Oatmeal (NOT instant)

Other grains (barley, couscous, quinoa)
Beans (black, pinto, kidney, chickpeas, etc.)
Fruits (apples, berries, oranges, pears, peaches, grapes, melons, etc.)
Nonfat yogurt
Whole wheat bread

Vegetables

Asparagus
Artichokes
Bell peppers (any color)
Broccol
Brussels sprouts
Cabbage
Carrots
Cauliflower

Celery
Cucumber
Green beans
Mushrooms
Onion
Spinach
Tomato
Zucchini

Stay tuned for the FREE DAY – you're going to LOVE it!!!

Water

We can hear the collective "Ughs" and we wish we could do something that would make this optional, but we can't and it's not. Water plays a key role in the metabolic process of the human body. Water makes up about 60 percent of your body weight. Every system and cell in your body depends on water for proper function. Water carries nutrients to your cells and organs and flushes toxins out of your body. When you don't drink enough water you feel sluggish and tired. Even mild dehydration can drain your energy and affect your performance.

Angie's Story: I'm not sure why I was so resistant to the concept of drinking water throughout the day, but I sure was!! When we were developing this program and Deb told me that I needed to be drinking a MINIMUM of 96 oz of water per day, plus an additional 16 oz per workout and, oh yeah, another 16 oz for each Grande Pikes Place coffee I consumed, I thought she was nuts! I had been taught by every other diet guru out there to drink 8 8-oz glasses of water per day – although I wasn't even drinking that much. But I was in "whatever it takes" mode and I was determined to make water consumption a habit. I armed myself with the tools I needed – a big 64 oz plastic jug filled with filtered water (which needed to be all gone before 5pm) and a 16 oz. glass for the office. The first day I was in the bathroom every 20 minutes I think. I thought I could hear myself "sloshing" when I walked across the room, but I drank it all. I drank 16 oz. in the morning with my vitamins, I drank another 16 oz with my workout, I drank 64 oz during the workday, another 16 oz during dinner – I thought I was going to spring a leak. A funny thing happened though. As the days passed, my skin started looking clearer and "glowy." I had more stamina for my workouts, more energy for work and life in general. The near constant low level headache that I had lived with for years was suddenly gone (huh, wonder if it was from dehydration). And hallelujah, I was suddenly "regular," – if you know what I mean.

That doesn't mean it was an easy habit to create. There were MANY days when Deb had to prod me about drinking my water, gave me the stink eye from across the office and pointed to my mostly full water jug, or thrust a glass in my hand as we passed in the hallway. Have I mentioned how awesome it is to have a live-in accountability partner? Now that drinking 100-125 oz of water each day is just a part of my life, I wonder how it is that I didn't shrivel up and blow away before – I mean I would go for DAYS without drinking any liquid besides coffee or tea!!

So, ditch the soda, the diet soda, the energy drinks, the sports drinks (unless you are using the right ones when you exercise) and DRINK YOUR WATER!!

- 16 oz when you wake up with your supplements (more on that in The Next Level)
- 16 oz with your workout
- 16 oz with each meal - breakfast, morning snack, lunch, afternoon snack and dinner
- An equivalent amount of water with every coffee or alcoholic beverage you consume (if you drink a Tall Starbucks, drink 12-oz of water; if you have a 6 oz. glass of wine with dinner, drink 6 extra ounces of water)

Helpful Hints to Keep You On Track

- Buy a 64 oz plastic jug and fill it each day and take it to work with you. Resolve to empty it before you leave the office each day.
- Set reminders in your Outlook calendar or on your phone so you remember to drink.
- If you sit down to eat, make sure you have a glass of water in front of you and don't get up from the table until it is all gone!

When Do I Eat?

As we have already established, you are going to eat 6 meals per day at approximately 3 hour intervals. Understand that the timing of your meals is critical! So, the natural question becomes "Okay, when does the clock start? How soon after waking up do I eat my first meal?" The answer depends on what you are doing upon waking. If you are waking up and getting the kids ready for school, getting yourself ready for work, playing on the internet, reading the newspaper – anything that does not require a great deal of physical exertion – you must eat your first meal within 30 minutes of waking. While you were sleeping your metabolism reduced to essentially the basal metabolic level – the level required to sustain and repair your body from the previous day's rigors. When you eat shortly after waking up in the morning your metabolism ramps back up for the day and continues to burn hot as you eat every few hours throughout the day. If you skip breakfast, or wait hours to eat, your metabolism stays at a very low level – which means you are burning calories at a very low level, which means you are not burning the fat off your body and that when you do finally eat, it is practically guaranteed that the majority of those calories will be stored as fat!

The exception to the 30 minute rule is if you work out first thing in the morning (more on the exercise part to come). That's us. We roll out of bed at 5:30 a.m. every weekday and head downstairs to our gym to work out. We do not eat before we exercise. According to a study published in *The Journal of Physiology (J Physiol. 2010 Nov 1;588(Pt 21):4289-302)*, exercising in a fasted state (usually possible only before breakfast), coaxes the body to burn a greater percentage of fat for fuel during vigorous exercise, instead of relying primarily on carbohydrates. Plus, the fat burning furnace continues even after your workout is complete. If you are exercising in the morning, maximize the fat-burning effectiveness by exercising on an empty stomach. If it is a cardio, interval training workout, then wait one hour after completing your workout before eating. If it is a weight lifting day, you want to consume a protein-rich meal (*we can't recommend meal replacement or protein shakes more highly – more on that*

91

to come) within 30 minutes of completing your workout. Then, space your meals in 3 hour intervals throughout the rest of the day. The exercise part is coming gang, hang in there.

Feed Your Body What It Needs At Bedtime

We've discussed how to eat when you wake up, now let's talk about the other end of the day – what should you eat for your last meal of the day before you go to bed at night? To answer this question, we need to take a very basic look at what your body is up to while you sleep. There are basically two phases of a person's sleep pattern – NREM (Non Rapid Eye Movement) sleep and REM(Rapid Eye Movement) sleep. An adult spends about 80% of sleeping hours in NREM sleep. During deep stages of NREM sleep, the body repairs and regenerates tissues, builds bone and muscle, and appears to strengthen the immune system. During REM sleep, brain activity is heightened and intense dreaming occurs. In this stage near muscle paralysis occurs (hence the recurring dream about not being able to move or scream in a stressful situation).

Your body requires the amino acids in proteins to facilitate the repair and regeneration that occur during NREM sleep. You can choose from any of the proteins on the *Release* Plan Endorsed Foods list and eat a serving of them before bed. For instance, you could have a cup of fat-free cottage cheese or two hard-boiled eggs, or some chicken breast or tuna – you just can't have the carbohydrate along with it (so a piece of boneless, skinless chicken breast would be fine, but a chicken sandwich would not work). Protein shakes offer a wonderfully convenient alternative to preparing and eating an actual meal at bedtime. Protein shakes provide a source of quality protein that will fuel your body's repair processes at a cellular level. The type of protein you use is up to you, there are all kinds of different formulations, including soy, whey, egg, casein protein, just to name a few. We have tried a LOT of different products by a lot of different manufacturers in a lot of different formulations, we have our favorite brand, but it is a very individual preference. We suggest that you look for a brand that has quality ingredients (not a list of unpronounceable chemicals), that tastes good, works well for you and is a good value. Protein shake mixes will give your body everthing it needs during its overnight regenerative phase.

The Free Day

Oh Free Day, how we love thee!!! The Free Day concept is not unique to our program. We first ran across it in Bill Phillips' wonderful book, *Body for Life* – and it has been a part of our nutritional program ever since! Here's the idea and then we'll give you the reasoning behind it.

The Free Day is one day each week when you get to rest and relax all the rules. You do not exercise and you not only have permission, but a physiological MANDATE to eat whatever you want on this one day. If you wake up with a hankering for chocolate cake (and we often do) then have it. Pizza? Eat the whole pie if you want to. Cheeseburger? Go for it – heck, have a double. Ice cream? Absolutely. Nothing is forbidden – eat what you want.

Angie's Story: Now, when I heard about the Free Day there were two phases to my reaction. For the first couple of months I could not bring myself to actually indulge fully in a free day. I might have some wine, but I didn't join Deb in chocolate cake for breakfast or eat big meals or anything. It was such a foreign concept and I was CERTAIN that if I indulged I would halt my progress, so I held back. But then my weight release stalled anyhow and Deb urged me to just enjoy myself that one day, so I did and my weight release resumed. Hmmmm... So then I went to the other extreme – how much food could I possibly pack into a free day without making myself throw up... and I would end up at the end of each Saturday feeling AWFUL!

I have finally reached a nice middle of the road with my free days (which are usually on Saturdays) – they go something like this:

7:00am	*Vanilla Meal Shake with skim milk, supplements*
8:00am	*Chocolate cake, coffee*
11:00am	*A healthy, delicious lunch – a Greek Chicken Pita Pizza or a wrap sandwich*
2:00pm	*Wheat thins and hummus*
3:00pm	*Starbucks (coffee or mocha or latte)*
5:00pm	*A lovely dinner – whatever we feel like – maybe seafood or a steak, maybe pizza, maybe burgers and onion rings and a couple of (or a few) glasses of red wine*
9:00pm	*Chocolate protein shake with skim milk*

It's generally somewhere between 2,500 and 4,000 calories, depending on the Saturday. The point is that I have what I want – if I've been craving something during the week, I will have it on my Free Day – PERIOD!!

Our daughter, on the other hand, eats until she is literally ill on her free day, but is very regimented during the other 6 days of the week and the weight comes off. It bears repeating, you have absolute permission to eat whatever you want on your free day, just make sure it spikes your calories to at least double what you normally eat.

How About a Free WEEK?

Here is where you are going to think we're **really** crazy, but stick with us for a second. We are suggesting that, every 4 months or so, you actually take a week off from your *Release* lifestyle – TOTALLY! Even if you feel like everything is going along just great, just take a vacation for 7 days – no exercise, 7 free days in a row. See, over time, your logic will creep up and you will start to feel like you are in a rut. The idea of having to work out 6 days per week (it's not what you think, keep reading) will feel burdensome and cravings might begin to kick in as Mr. X rears his ugly head and asks "Why should you only have one free day a week – I want more…" Forever is a long time and Mr. X will reach up and grab you and tell you that you just can't keep doing this. So you let him win for a week every 4 months and you give yourself permission to be a couch potato and watch TV all day and eat whatever you want and sleep til noon – whatever your version of slug heaven is. What you'll find is that you've actually created a new paradigm that craves the proper food and exercise and you'll find that you can't wait until Monday morning to get back to "normal.". The free week can be a great reminder of what life was like before your *Release* program, and a fabulous motivator to get back to it when the week is over.

Aside from the psychological break, physically OVER training can be an issue as well. Deb especially notices overtraining symptoms – all of a sudden workouts are more difficult and less effective; she starts to experience insomnia and extreme fatigue. So, every 4-ish months (for us it's normally the week between Christmas and New Years, the week after Easter and a week in August), we take a complete week off from meal plans and exercise. The free week makes planning for holidays and summer vacation really easy! But you know, a funny thing happens about 3-4 days into the free week… we start craving a workout and would pretty much kill for a piece of chicken and a sweet potato!!

Deb Cheslow & Angie Flynn

CHAPTER EIGHT

OVERCOMING OBJECTIONS

In this chapter, we would like to address some of the most common objections we hear when it comes to the *Release* Plan. Unfortunately, a large percentage of the population has a real difficulty with change. The fact is this: If you want your life to change, you have to change your life. It's so simple and so obvious and yet far too many people will allow their logic to throw up objections that will derail their progress.

This is CRAZY! How Can it Possibly Work?

Here's the science behind the Free Day in *very* basic terms...

Our bodies are the product of millions of years of miraculous evolution – natural selection, survival of the fittest. Our ancestors lived in caves and had to hunt and gather their food on a daily basis because it wouldn't stay fresh and edible for any meaningful length of time. When food was readily available (the animals weren't hibernating or migrating and various fruits and vegetables were in season), our ancestors' metabolism burned high and they were lean and agile to allow them to chase, catch and kill the animals that they ate for food or to forage through the underbrush for berries or climb trees to gather fruit. When the seasons changed and fall deepened into winter, food became scarcer. Our ancestors' metabolisms depressed and they built up layers of fat to feed/fuel their bodies during the coming winter when there was precious little to eat and their greatest physical activity was shivering in the cold of their caves. Then spring would come again, the snow would melt, the animals would return and the cycle would begin again.

Today, even though the vast majority of us don't have to worry about a lack of food in any season, our bodies react much the same way. If we eat high quality food and use our bodies physically on a regular basis, our metabolism stays ramped at a high level. However, if we start restricting calories and/or stop moving our bodies there is an evolutionary switch that flips inside that says "Whoa, hold up there! Winter is coming!" and our metabolic fire dies down to barely an ember. This can happen in as little as a week! Is it any wonder that we have an obesity problem when we give our bodies every possible physical signal that "it's winter" (no physical activity) so that our metabolisms plummet and then we sit around stuffing our faces with super-sized fast food meals? The disconnect seems abundantly clear!!

Let's look at a typical low calorie diet for a minute. Let's assume that you eat 1,000 calories per day and you burn an average of 300 calories through exercise, 3 days per week and you sustain this for several weeks. Now, if you are a 45 year old woman who weighs 145 lbs and is 5'5" tall, you require approximately 1,550 calories per day just to keep your heart beating, your lungs pumping and your cells multiplying (using the Harris-Benedict equation for calculating basal metabolic rate). At a net 871 calories per day $[(3 \times 300)/7 = 129$ calories burned by exercise daily on average. 1,000 calories consumed - 129 calories burned = 871 net calorie intake per day], you are at a caloric deficit. You are literally not eating enough calories to stay alive over the long haul. So your body needs to "find" the extra calories it needs and reduce what it requires for sustenance – the calories your body requires to breathe, digest, excrete, regulate your body temperature, perform tissue maintenance or cell renewal and so on.

Here's where insult gets added to injury. Your body will certainly pull some fuel from fat on a low-calorie diet, but it will also pull just as much from muscle mass (which is metabolically active) causing that gaunt, wasted look that people get when they have been on a crash diet. In conjunction with losing some fat and muscle, your metabolism also depresses – causing you to be able to maintain your bodily systems on fewer and fewer calories. Here's the double whammy part... When you inevitably go off your diet (because, HELLO, you're STARVING to death) and binge – or even resume eating the way you did before your diet, you will gain weight because you've killed your metabolism. And you won't gain back the muscle you lost, you gain it all back as fat. This is why yo-yo dieters just seem to get fatter and fatter over time. They kill their metabolism by severely restricting their calories and making their bodies think it's winter and there's a famine and they cannibalize their body's fat burning muscle! Then they go back to eating "normally" and instead of just maintaining their weight, they gain weight. So here it is, plain and simple: *YOU WILL ALWAYS GAIN WEIGHT OVER THE LONG TERM BY DIETING! ALWAYS!!*

The *Release* Plan's Free Day provides insurance against this evolutionary "famine" switch getting tripped. Although not a "low calorie diet" by any stretch of the imagination, the *Release* Plan does create a calorie deficit (you are, on net, burning more calories through exercise and normal bodily functions than you are consuming) each week. If you break down the *Release* Meal Plan, you will find that each day's calorie total is between 1,500 and 2,500 (depending on if you're a woman or a man). Allowing yourself that one day each week where you eat far more calories than you would on the other six days of the week reassures your body that it is indeed still springtime and food is plentiful – no need to shut down the metabolism. It is a situation where eating MORE on that one day will actually result in your continued weight loss – **without destroying your metabolic furnace and without cannibalizing your muscle mass!** It is insurance against the dreaded weight release plateau!

And to make it even better, there are other psychic benefits to the Free Day!

1. It's a great cravings-buster because you are never more than 6 days from your next free day when you have the freedom to indulge whatever craving you have – nothing is forbidden;
2. It promotes an "abundance" mindset. So often when we are "dieting" we feel deprived – there are constant feelings of lack and limitation. Angie rarely went out with friends when she was hardcore dieting because she couldn't stand to sit there and eat salad with no dressing and drink water with lemon while her friends were having buffalo chicken wings and beer. The free day does away with that because you can schedule your social calendar around that day and have whatever you want!

3. After a free day, you are much more likely to jump right back on your *Release* Plan for the week because you have satisfied your cravings.
4. When you do have your favorite foods, they actually taste BETTER and you enjoy them more!

We love our free day and know you will too. Don't be afraid of it. Play with the day until you find the balance between eating like it's a regular day and stuffing yourself until you throw up - find what works for you – and it might be different from week to week. Sometimes our free day doesn't look all that much different than a regular day except that we eat MORE of what we would usually eat (to double the calories) and perhaps add in a few glasses of wine and a some chocolate – other weeks it a veritable food orgy!!! This is a LIFESTYLE, not something you are going to do for a fixed period of time and then stop because it's "over."

The free day gives you freedom, choice and control. People often ask if they can change what day of the week they have their free day on from week to week. Yes, you can, but be careful. You are forming new habits and the repetition of patterns of behavior is very important, so try to stick with the same day each week. BUT, that said, this is a lifestyle, not a prison, and LIFE HAPPENS, so if you have an event that you would like to be free to eat whatever you choose then go for it. Or, if you find yourself in a situation where you didn't plan correctly and end up having a food binge or something, don't beat yourself up – take the day as your free day and move on. What you can't do (or SHOULDN'T do) is have your free day for this week on Saturday and then decide to have next week's free day on Sunday (the very next day). Remember, your body needs a "reminder" every 7 days or so that "it's springtime" and that there is no need to shut down the metabolism to survive the long winter ahead.

How am I Supposed to Cook Six Meals Per Day EVERY Day?

That's a very reasonable question and one we struggled with as well. It's hard enough some days to get three meals on the table, much less SIX! But trust us, it's just a matter of adjusting your paradigms regarding the definition of a meal. Think for a moment what images the term "meal" brings to your mind. Do you see a picture of a huge plate of food served in multiple courses? Well, that's not what we're talking about here. A *Release* Plan meal consists of a portion of protein, a portion of carbohydrates, a glass of water and a veggie thrown in a couple of times per day.

We are incredibly busy people, we do not have a chef on staff, and we go out to eat at restaurants very rarely – we prepare our own meals every day, just like you do – and we prepare SIX of them every day! How? We follow a three step success plan:

1. Planned menus
2. Drink at least two meals
3. Cook once, eat twice (or thrice)

Step 1 – Planning: Every Friday, Angie plans our menu for the upcoming week. Groceries are bought and prepped so that meals can be quickly prepared. Generally, we will plan two different breakfast, lunch and afternoon snack options for the week and three different dinner options. 90% of the meals we make can be prepared in less than 30 minutes and most of our daytime meals need to be portable so we can take them on the road with us as we meet with clients.

Step 2 – Drink at least two meals: We have nutrition shakes for our first and last meals of the day – a meal replacement shake in the morning and a protein shake before bed. These shakes are AMAZING!! They are quick and easy (1 or 2 scoops of powder in 8 ounces of skim milk, shake and go) and give your body exactly what it needs! The meal replacement shake offers the same nutritional profile as a piece of chicken, a baked potato and a cup of broccoli! And the protein shake is just that – pure protein, no carbs and no fat!

There are many different brands of replacement shakes available in nutrition and health food stores, that are nourishing, convenient, quick to prepare, portable, delicious and really do keep you satisfied for hours. The meal shake we prefer also contains an amino acid called *leucine* that protects against muscle loss as you release weight from your body (so the weight you release is actually from fat, not muscle). Before bed we have a protein shake so that, as discussed earlier, our bodies have adequate protein to facilitate the rebuilding and regeneration of our bodies during the night.

Like we said, there are dozens of brands and formulations of protein and meal replacement shakes available on the market today. We'll be honest with you, there are some NASTY shake mixes out there! To find the best combination of taste, nutrition, performance and value feel free to experiment on your own, or contact us at release@myreleaseplan.com for some specific recommendations.

When you are deciding which shake mix to incorporate into your lifestyle check the following:

- Make sure there is adequate protein (at least 15 grams per serving)
- Balanced carbohydrates (roughly equal to the amount of protein)
- Low in sugar (but not full of a bunch of artificial sweeteners either)
- Low fat
- Read the ingredients – how far can you read before you can't pronounce the words - you don't want to be pouring chemicals down your throat!
- Great taste – if you are going to consume something, shouldn't it taste good?

There are ALL KINDS of surprising ways to blend the shakes into a deliciously decadent treat – like a Dreamsicle Shake, an Iced Chai Latte, Apple Pie ala Mode and more. We have included several shake recipes in the Meal Planning section, but you can find dozens more at *www.MyReleasePlan.com*.

Do you have to incorporate shakes into your meal plan? Absolutely not. You can just replace the shakes with 2 more protein/carbohydrate/vegetable meals. We LOVE the shakes because they are quick, convenient, portable and fit into our lives very easily, but it is not mandatory that you use them in your meal plan.

Step 3 – Cook once, eat twice (or thrice): When we prepare a recipe we double or triple it so we can have multiple meals ready to go from each cooking session. We INSIST on having family dinners whenever possible (and we usually succeed in all gathering around the dinner table 5-6 nights per week), but with all of our various schedules it would be next to impossible if we had to cook a full meal every single night. So, we cook once and then reheat leftovers the next night (or plan to have the leftovers for lunch the next day).

In reality, you will likely GAIN time in your schedule following the *Release* Plan because of the planning aspect and the cook once, eat twice philosophy.

Let's quickly recap… You get to eat more often … Feel better … *Release* weight … Have more energy … AND, gain extra time in your schedule… This has to be sounding pretty great so far, right? Well, the good news is that the best is yet to come, so read on!

The Shakes Taste Terrible

Our question is what brand of shake are you using? There is no doubt that meal replacement shakes are an acquired taste, but there is a HUGE variation in taste across brands. We have tried a lot of different shake mixes and premade shakes and some are truly awful – to the point where we threw the whole canister away rather than drink another one. In the beginning, use some of the shake recipes in this book or on *MyReleasePlan.com*. They are really delicious! We are always happy to offer specific product recommendations - just drop us a note at release@myreleaseplan.com.

This Sounds Expensive – I'm on a Budget!

Now we come to the inevitable question, "But, isn't it expensive?" There are a few ways to answer this question, but the end result is the same, "NO!" Let's break down the cost issue:

1.   The Shakes: At first glance adding two different types of shakes to your eating plan may appear costly, but if you do the math, the price an "expensive" meal replacement shake is ~$3.25/shake and a protein shake is ~$1.40/shake. We submit that you couldn't go to McDonald's and get whatever greasy breakfast special du jour they were serving up for less than $3.25 and what bed time snack do you know of that costs less than $1.40?

2.   Whole foods: You will notice that the *Release* Plan contains very little processed or packaged food. You are fueling your body with REAL food – meats, eggs, cheeses, fruits, vegetables, whole grains and it may set off budgetary alarms, but we can tell you from personal experience that your grocery bill (and the time you spend in the food store) may actually DECREASE when you begin following the *Release* Plan. You are going to find that you become a perimeter shopper. You will spend 95% of the time you are in the food store in the outer regions of the store – the produce section, the dairy section, the meat and seafood counter, the freezer section – making quick trips into the interior aisles for bread, pasta, rice, tuna and very little else! For all of their supposed convenience, all that processed, boxed "food" that is currently filling your shopping cart is pricey!

Angie's Story: Before I began eating this way, I was spending about $150/week at the food store to feed my family of 3 (and that didn't count all of the $20 pop ins I made during the week to grab something on a whim) and we ate like crap, quite frankly! After I started the plan, I was still shopping once per week, my family size had increased to 5 people and I was spending an average of ~$230/week, so on a per person basis, my grocery bill actually DECREASED!!

Now, if you are currently sustaining yourself on Ramen Noodles and boxed Macaroni and Cheese then, yes, your grocery bill is going to increase, but what you've been doing isn't working – the food you have been fueling your body with isn't giving you the results you want, and that brings us to point #3.

3. What's your health worth? What is your current monthly expenditure for prescription drugs (high blood pressure medicine, cholesterol lowering drugs, pain killers, sleep aids, indigestion medicines, laxatives, etc.)? How many times per year do you get sick and have to go to the doctor or miss work? Check out Deb's story:

In 1997, I had half my thyroid removed because of a suspicious cyst (which turned out to be benign). The doctors told me that the remaining half would function fine, but mine did not. I was put on a drug that was a synthetic version of the thyroid hormone produced by a normal thyroid gland and was told I would be on it for the rest of my life. Then in 2001, I found that when I would ride the bike I would have a tingling and a numbing sensation in my legs once in a while and sometimes at night when I would watch TV with my girls I couldn't get comfortable. Over time these episodes became more frequent and more intense. I became aware that several of my friends had developed Multiple Sclerosis and I couldn't get it out of my head that maybe I had it too. After my husband and I separated, I needed sleeping pills to sleep thru the night. See, in my mind everything I wanted and had built in my life had walked out the door.

I was miserable – I threw the grandest pity party the world has ever seen. All my energy was directed at how horrible my life was and what my husband had done to me. By summer 2004 the restless leg symptoms were so bad, I couldn't get comfortable sitting at my desk at work; I couldn't sleep at night. The only way to get relief was through exercise. I went to the medical community for help. I saw doctors and neurologists and tried drug after drug. Some helped, some had side-effects that were even worse than the RLS, but all lost their efficacy over time. My body was like a sponge and kept adjusting to the dosages, so drug after drug was eliminated as I maxed out the allowable dosage.

Then my neurologist suggested I start taking an anti-anxiety medication which I was vehemently opposed to – I wasn't depressed (yeah, right)!! He literally told me to put the stigma aside and "get over it"; that there was nothing wrong with taking anti-depressants/anti-anxiety medication; "everybody's doing it," but he also said it could help the RLS. So, here I was on drugs for my thyroid, on antidepressants, and one dosage increase away from maxing out the last known RLS drug on the market!! I couldn't function without the medications, even though the side-effects made life miserable. We were running out of drugs to try. I was scared! My RLS symptoms were getting worse. I was lonelier than I had even been. I hated my job. I hated my life. I really believed that at 38 years old the best of life was behind me.

As you can read in "The Next Level" chapter, I was introduced to a line of natural products about this time and I added meal replacement and soy protein shakes to my nutritional plan, along with some basic supplements. The products were the vehicle for my belief and in an incredibly short period of time (about 3 months) I was feeling better than I had in years. My doctors weaned me off all of the drugs I was on (except for the thyroid medication) and released me with a clean bill of health.

Then in August, 2008 I became aware of a new product that was promoted as an anti-aging tonic (the literature said it actually repaired and renewed at the DNA level). I went to my doctor and told him that I wanted him to monitor me as I weaned myself off my thyroid medication, somehow KNOWING that I had healed my thyroid. He lectured me about how dangerous that was, but I was determined. I went in for blood tests periodically to check my thyroid levels, and by November, I had a perfectly normal blood panel and my doctor was dumbfounded – to the point of asking me to come in for a repeat blood test *because the results that were sitting in front of him did not seem possible. I have been off the thyroid medication since August, 2008 and in May, 2012 I had a complete blood panel run; at 47 years old my stats are pegged in the normal range.*

I now know that I was an "unconscious competent" in this material throughout my life – I created my health, then I destroyed it and then I rebuilt it again.

Now, we are not promising medical miracles, but it is a fact that many of the most prevalent ailments that people suffer from can be alleviated by creating a strong, healthy body! Except for routine preventative screenings, we have not been to the doctor in years, saving us thousands of dollars in medical bills, prescription costs and lost time at work – those are the kinds of results that you CAN have on the *Release* Plan!

The bottom line is that the lifestyle you currently live is a paradigm – just the same as the way you brush your teeth or whether you put your right leg into your pants first or your left – it's habit, it's comfortable. Making a change will be uncomfortable and take concentrated effort. Remember, half of getting what you want lies in knowing what you have to give up to get it. Giving up habits that aren't working for you and replacing them with new habits that will carry you where you want to go may take some effort, but it is so worth it!

I Could NEVER Give Up...

Good!! The *Release* Plan will NEVER ask you to give up any of your favorite foods or drinks! You can have ANYTHING you want on your Free Day – you are never more than 7 days away from that which you desire most. It's not what you do all the time that gets you the results you want; it's what you do MOST of the time that counts. No one is perfect and we all have our culinary vices – Deb's is chocolate and Angie's is wine. We limit those foods to our Free Days. Again, this is a lifestyle, not a prison!

A Note About Alcohol

Although we suggest that alcohol should be a Free Day item, studies indicate that red wine can be beneficial to your health. There is an antioxidant in red wine – a polyphenol called resveratrol – that has been shown to protect blood vessels and arteries from damage by decreasing LDL (bad) cholesterol. There is also research evidence that suggests resveratrol reduces the risk of inflammation and blood clotting, both of which can lead to heart disease. While we do not encourage anyone who does not already drink wine to start consuming it, if you DO enjoy having a glass of wine occasionally (and you can just have one glass), the *Release* Plan certainly allows for a 6 oz. glass of red wine 2-3 days per week. However, beer and liquor should be reserved for Free Days only.

CHAPTER NINE

What Do I Eat If... Help for Sticky Situations

This section is designed to give you some ideas for handling situations that pop up in life all the time that can be big derailers on a normal "diet." It's really quite easy to stay on plan when you're in complete control of everything you're eating 100% of the time; you know, when you're the one choosing the foods you're going to eat, and the one preparing those foods, and the one ensuring that the portion sizes are correct at all times. When you can do this 24 hours a day, 7 days a week, sticking to your plan really isn't difficult at all. Unfortunately for most of us, this just isn't reality. In the real world, life tends to get in the way of our ideal eating habits on a fairly regular basis. Understand clearly that the *Release* Plan is not about perfection (and we have a great example coming up that illustrates the point beautifully) – this IS real life AND you are on your journey to a new LIFESTYLE, not a 2 month, 4 month or 1 year program that you endure and then comes to an end. It's what you do MOST of the time that will lead you to the results you want, hence the Free Day (and Free Week) concept. So, how do you handle:

- The unanticipated meal at a restaurant;
- The church (club, school, neighborhood, etc.) potluck dinner;
- The business lunch;
- Happy hour?

First of all, you have a trump card in your pocket in the Free Day, so if you find yourself blindsided by a situation where you HAVE to eat and there is NOTHING that will work for a *Release* Plan meal, you can throw this card and have your Free Day and enjoy yourself. That option is always available to you as long as you haven't already had your Free Day that week. We personally don't like doing this, because we like to plan our Free Day for maximum enjoyment (notice we didn't say "maximum quantity") and, we don't know about you, but Sally Muckenfuch's Chicken ala King Surprise at the church potluck is not worth blowing our Free Day over (sorry Sally).

The Unanticipated Restaurant Meal

It's 6pm and your significant other picks you up from work unexpectedly and whisks you off to a restaurant for dinner or you are out running errands and you have 2 hours longer to go and you forgot to bring your food with you and you're ravenous. Regardless of the reason, you find yourself sitting at a table in a restaurant with a menu opened in front of you. What do you order? Restaurant menus seem to offer an endless list of one fat-laden, calorie bomb after another. One thing we like to do is order an appetizer – like a shrimp cocktail – and a side salad. Or, believe it or not, you can always order **off** the menu. We do this often and restaurants are happy to accommodate – order a piece of grilled or broiled chicken or fish (no butter please), a baked potato or baked sweet potato or serving of rice, and a steamed vegetable. This is a PERFECT *Release* Plan meal!

Now, restaurant portion sizes are out of control so also ask for a to-go box when you're ordering. That way when they bring your meal, you can measure out your "fist" of carb and your "palm" of protein and scoop the rest in the to-go container and take it home for tomorrow's lunch! PERFECT! Getting everything off your plate except the portion that you are eating does a couple of beneficial things: First, you only have what you're supposed to eat on your plate (no opportunity for mindless nibbling during your conversation). Second, huge restaurant portions work in your favor from a value perspective, giving you one or two additional meals in your to-go box, saving you time (you don't have to cook) and money!!

The Potluck Dinner

The best thing about a potluck dinner is that everyone brings something, so that means YOU brought something too. Just bring a dish that is plan friendly and eat that – simple!

The Business Lunch

We're not big fans of business lunches – there's something about trying to close a deal and chew at the same time that doesn't work for us, so we generally just don't. However, there are many people who love meeting over lunch. The nice thing about a business lunch meeting is that in 99% of the cases it is pre-arranged. When we know we are eating out, we like to see if the restaurant has an online version of their menu available (most restaurants do these days) and we plans our meals in advance. If you make your decisions in advance it's a lot easier to stick with the plan – you don't even need a menu because you already know what you plan to order. If there are no good options on the menu, then you can always order off-menu like you did in the first example. Remember that to-go box – even lunch portions at restaurants can be too big. You can also eat one of your meals just before your lunch meeting and then order water or iced tea and a side salad at the restaurant (the vegetable component of the meal you just ate).

Happy Hour

It's 5pm and your best friend just called complaining that s/he hasn't seen you in forever and wants to meet for a drink to catch up. What do you do? Assuming you want to meet up with your friend, GO! Having one light beer or one glass of wine is not going to wreck your day! But limit yourself to one drink. Caveat… We have seen many a good intention go the way of the dinosaur when alcohol is involved. Do yourself a favor – even if you have to stop at the corner 7-11 and grab an apple and a couple of pieces of string cheese – eat something before you go.

In summary, the *Release* Plan is designed to be a very flexible lifestyle that you can adapt within certain guidelines to work with life as it happens. Sometimes it takes being a little creative; sometimes you have to ask for what you want if you don't see it; sometimes a little preplanning is involved, but you can absolutely manage your *Release* Plan and still live in the outside world.

Deb Cheslow & Angie Flynn

CHAPTER TEN

In Pursuit of Perfection: A Case Study

We hear it all the time – "I blew my diet out of the water today, there is no hope for me, I may as well just give up." This is hogwash!!! While it may hold that the stricter you follow your eating and exercise plan, the faster you will achieve your goal, it is not true that you need to be "perfect" in every moment of every day to get where you want to go! First of all, "perfect" is unattainable – if perfect is what you're striving for, then you will continually be disappointed. Some days you may think you get close to "perfect," but, of course, there is no such thing. "Did I really put 100% into my workout?" "Could I have pushed myself a little (or a lot) harder?" "Were my meals perfectly spaced?" "Was that piece of chicken the perfect size?" These are questions your authors ask themselves all the time and over and over again, and the answer is "NO, I didn't even approach "perfect," BUT I am still moving toward my goal."

Here is a case in point:

Angie's Story: Let me tell you a story that illustrates so many important points and it actually happened to me "YESTERDAY!" "Yesterday" was February 5, 2012 when Deb and I took our daughter, Nicki, and two of her friends to Universal Studios Islands of Adventure in Orlando to celebrate her 17th birthday. It was also the day before Deb's birthday, so we were all in a celebratory mood. Deb and I chose to have our "free" day the day before. Our rationale was that theme park food is usually not all that great and we'd be so busy riding rides and shopping in the shops that we wouldn't have time to really enjoy a restaurant anyhow. Hmmm, probably should have researched a little better. If you've been to the Universal parks you of course know about the CityWalk section, which has (among other things), not one but TWO Emeril Lagasse restaurants – Emeril's and Tchoup Chop - Jimmy Buffet's Margaritaville, Hard Rock Café, etc., not to mention Starbucks!!!! We found ourselves in a fabulous food and drink Mecca and we had a backpack filled with protein bars, 2 salmon cakes and water. NOOOOOOOOOOOOO!!!!!! Oh well, live and learn, we'll know better next time, right? Wellllll, not exactly.

*In our family there are several days per year that count as extra free days if you want to claim them – Thanksgiving Day, Christmas Eve and Christmas Day, New Year's Day and your birthday. Deb was covered – she could take the day as her birthday free day if she found something that she really wanted, but I needed to make a decision. I needed to decide whether I was going to walk the straight and narrow and stick to my food plan whether or not Deb strayed or that I would enjoy the day without restrictions as well. We were walking to the first ride of the day (in the Wizarding World of Harry Potter – which, by the way, was **very** cool) and we had this very discussion and I kind of made the decision not to decide. I decided that I would stick to my food plan, UNLESS some opportunity for something really extraordinary or fun came along, because I didn't want my vibration (which was sky high) to be dampened by feelings of lack and limitation. Surprisingly, Deb accepted my indecision (a VERY rare occurrence) and we continued with the day. So, here's what happened...*

We went to the Hog's Head Tavern around lunch tine and they had all kinds of fun things on the menu – Cornish pasties, turkey legs, shepherd's pie and more – but what I WANTED was the rotisserie chicken salad and to try Butterbeer (hey, we were in Harry Potter World – you HAVE to try the butterbeer!!!). So, that's what I had (Deb too) and it was delicious and I was quite satisfied!! The butterbeer was interesting – like cream soda with vanilla-mashmallow whipped cream on top. It was very sweet and we both only had 2-3 sips of it before enough was enough. Think about that for a second. Deb and I gave ourselves permission to splurge and we both wanted a salad with grilled chicken on top. Go figure... maybe there really is something to this "paradigm" stuff afterall!

Around 2:30 we were both hungry again and each had one of the protein bars we brought with us while people watching in Seuss Landing.

Then at 4:30 we were both STARVING. We had exhausted the gift shops and decided to head over to the CityWalk section and see what was there. We ended up, ironically, on the Porch of Indecision at Jimmy Buffet's Margaritaville. Deb had a frozen drink and I had a glass of wine and we shared the peel and eat shrimp and the Crab, Shrimp and Mushroom Dip appetizers. We sat for a long time – the weather was picture perfect and we savored the food and drink. It was delicious and PERFECT!!! We talked and laughed and had the best time.

Then we topped the day off with a coffee at Starbucks – nothing fancy, just a regular coffee.

Lessons I learned from this exercise:

1. *Deb and I had the best time EVER, so while I was not "perfect" as far as my food plan was concerned, it sure did FEEL like the PERFECT day!!!*
2. *I was able to maintain an incredibly high vibration all day long because I was in an abundant frame of mind – I knew that if I rounded a corner and found something I really wanted, I could have it. I was never operating from a mindset of lack or limitation. The choices I made were what I WANTED, not what I thought I SHOULD have – and yet, they were great choices (okay, the butterbeer and the dip were definitely out of bounds, but I had what I wanted and threw the rest away).*

Helpful Hint: The Clean Plate Club

Are you a member of the "clean plate club?" Did your parents glower at you and talk about the starving children in Africa if you left food on your plate when you were growing up? Guess what – THAT is a paradigm!! Why on earth would you be so averse to "wasting food" knowing you would make yourself sick trying to eat it all? If you are indeed a member of the "clean plate club," try an experiment for 30 days: Always leave a little food on your plate. You may have heard this one before, but believe it or not it actually works! Not only are you consuming less calories over a period of time by doing this at every meal, but you are also giving yourself some positive reinforcement. You will feel much better when you feel as if you didn't just eat your meal "like a pig" but like a real civilized person. It will also simply reinforce your positive actions towards weight release each time you push your plate away with a little food left on it. That simple action empowers you with a feeling of abundance – you didn't have to eat it all. And, while we're at it, let's be real, that food you leave on your plate is not going to help the starving children of the world – it's either going in the trash or it's going in you. And you being unhealthy is not going to help anyone!

---

3. *I discovered that I would rather have a little bit of something wonderful than a whole lot of something mediocre.*

4. *When I got home and journaled what I had eaten during the day, I was surprised to find that I had actually consumed fewer (net) calories than I usually do when I am ON plan (because of all the hours of walking we did at the park)!*

5. *I was extra motivated to get up on Monday morning and have a fantastic workout and launch into a great week.*

    We will say it over and over again, every day you are trading your LIFE for what you do. Life is to be lived with gusto! What good is it to set a goal of reaching your ideal weight and fitness level if you aren't allowed to live FULLY while you're on the journey? I can promise you that if I had decided to stick to my plan – no matter what – yesterday, by the end of the day I would have been ready to sell my first born child for a French fry. All the smells from the vendors at the park would have had me positively ravenous and I would have been miserable. My vibration would have taken a nose dive and I would be further from my goals today because of it. LIFE HAPPENS!!! There are going to be all sorts of things that will pop up and derail you from your best intentions. In those moments it is crucial that you look at the situation holistically. By that I mean, what's going to happen to your overall mindset if you take a particular course of action and, in the end, will it move you toward or away from your end goal? I honestly believe that I am CLOSER to my goal because of my "cheat" yesterday than I would be if I had rigidly followed my plan. Now, that said, will I go downstairs after I finish typing this and gorge myself on chocolate ice cream because I like ice cream? NO, of course not. The difference is that freeing my mind from the worry of every bite I was putting in my mouth yesterday enhanced my day. There would be NOTHING positive about raiding the ice cream shelf while sitting here alone. Every bite would take my vibration lower instead of higher.

CAVEAT: No "Cheating" for the First 30 Days - PERIOD

The question you need to ask yourself is this: What is your HABIT? What do you do, day in and day out, with only the rarest exception? Is "cheating" the habit or the rare exception? It takes 30 days to build a new habit, so there can be NO "CHEATS" during that first 30 days as you retrain your brain to habitualize the *Release* Plan as your eating lifestyle.

Deb Cheslow & Angie Flynn

This is where an accountability partner can be very helpful. Deb and I talked about the decision we made yesterday at length and analyzed what the best course of action was and afterwards we talked about it some more and teased out all the lessons that had come out of the day.

CHAPTER ELEVEN

Advance Decision Making

Let's talk for a little bit about decision making. Are you good at making decisions? Most people aren't; in fact, if you are like 97% of people out there you probably HATE making decisions and were never really taught HOW to make them. Decision making is certainly not taught in school and yet it is without a doubt the most important skill a person can have when it comes to improving their life. If you think about it, most people are very indecisive – either they put off making decisions or they just ask other people for THEIR opinion on the matter and then make a decision based upon the collective input they receive. That is no way to go through life. Indecision causes disintegration – you are either creating or disintegrating, nothing stands still. You are either moving forward or you are going backwards – status quo is a myth- it doesn't exist. The most effective people out there are those who make decisions right where they are with the information they have in the moment. They commit to their decision and are unlikely to change their mind without great deliberation. If you study people who are really good at making decisions, you'll find that they all possess another wonderful quality – self-confidence. They believe they can do, have or be anything they set their minds to – failure doesn't really enter into the equation. And if they do fail they shrug it off quickly and keep moving forward. So, let us ask you a question… Are you HOPING this program will work for you or have you DECIDED that it will? There's a tremendous difference. Hoping leads to guaranteed failure while a committed decision leads to guaranteed success. Think about it, what would your life be like if every time you said, "I should…," you DID?

Anytime you need to make a decision, there are four questions you need to ask yourself:

1. Do I want to be, to do or to have this?
2. Will being, doing or having this move me in the direction of my goals?
3. Is being, doing or having this in harmony with God's laws or the laws of the universe?

4. Will being, doing or having this violate the rights of others?

If you answer "Yes" to questions 1-3 and "No" to question 4, then you make your decision right where you are with what you have!

When planning a trip, what is the first thing you do? You make reservations with the airline, the hotel, the rental car company, etc., so that you can get to your destination hassle free and have your accommodations waiting for you, right? We don't know about you, but we would find it incredibly stressful to wake up on the day of a trip, knowing that we needed to be in San Diego by dinner time and just HOPE that we could get a seat on a plane and have a place to sleep in San Diego when we got there. No, you don't do that. You make decisions about your journey before you ever take the first step of the trip. You also don't buy your ticket to San Diego and then get to the airport and see all the other nifty destinations that you could go to and throw your ticket to San Diego in the trash and go to Omaha instead, even though your hotel, your rental car, your family, friends and the convention you need to attend are all in San Diego!! Why shouldn't you employ this same technique – advance decision making - when it comes to your weight release journey? Think about it, if you DECIDE that, come what may, you will only eat foods that are on your eating plan, then it doesn't matter that you walk into a meeting and your host has laid out an all-you-can-eat chocolate buffet – you've already made your decision. Unless "all-you-can-eat chocolate" has somehow made it onto your daily menu, you've made an advance decision not to eat it! Making decisions in advance can solve so many problems and take the guesswork or surprise out of things! You are holding your ticket to your ideal body in your hands – don't just throw it in the trash when something seemingly more attractive comes along.

Ideas for employing Advance Decision Making in your *Release* Plan:

1. Plan your menu for the upcoming week and prepare meals in advance, so you can brown bag. If you have food that you

know you can take with you, you'll be much less likely to eat something that is off your plan;

2. Plan your exercise calendar each week – know when and where you are going to exercise and what you are going to do each day. When you know what you need to do and when you need to do it, you will be much less likely to find an excuse to skip your workout.

3. If you know you are going to an event that will be serving food that you can't eat, let the host know that you won't be eating – or just go and don't eat – chances are very good that no one will even notice. Trust us; we do it all the time and haven't insulted or offended anyone yet!

Deb Cheslow & Angie Flynn

CHAPTER TWELVE

Time to Move It!

Let's go back to a theme from the first section of this book - Information vs. Action – Knowing vs. Doing. It really is a no-brainer that we should include some physical exercise in our daily lives. We all KNOW we should, but so many of us – despite our very best intentions don't DO it. We KNOW exercise is good for us, but we FEEL like sleeping in or watching re-runs of *Two and a Half Men*. According to the Mayo Clinic, regular exercise benefits us in a whole variety of ways.

1. Exercise controls weight: Duh. Exercise can help prevent excess weight gain or help maintain weight release. When you engage in physical activity, you burn calories. When you burn more calories than you take in through food/beverage, you will release weight. Pure and simple.

2. Exercise combats adverse health conditions and diseases: No matter what your current weight, being active boosts high-density lipoprotein (HDL), or "good," cholesterol and decreases unhealthy triglycerides. This one-two punch keeps your blood flowing smoothly, which decreases your risk of cardiovascular diseases. In fact, regular physical activity can help you prevent or manage a wide range of health problems and concerns, including stroke, metabolic syndrome, type 2 diabetes, depression, certain types of cancer, arthritis and falls.

3. Exercise improves mood: Physical activity stimulates various brain chemicals that may leave you feeling happier and more relaxed. You may also feel better about your appearance and yourself when you exercise regularly, which can boost your confidence and improve your self-esteem. So, before you head to the doctor for a prescription for an anti-depressant, try going for a walk!

4. Exercise boosts energy: Regular physical activity can improve your muscle strength and boost your endurance. Exercise and physical activity deliver oxygen and nutrients to your tissues

and help your cardiovascular system work more efficiently. And when your heart and lungs work more efficiently, you have more energy to go about your daily chores. People continually use the excuse that they don't have time to exercise, but in reality exercise gives you MORE TIME in your schedule because you have so much more energy and can accomplish so much more each day!

5. Exercise promotes better sleep: Regular physical activity can help you fall asleep faster and deepen your sleep. Just don't exercise too close to bedtime, or you may be too energized to fall asleep.

6. Exercise puts the spark back into your sex life: Aww Yeah!! Regular physical activity can leave you feeling energized and looking better, which may have a positive effect on your sex life. But there's more to it than that. Regular physical activity can lead to enhanced arousal for women. And men who exercise regularly are less likely to have problems with erectile dysfunction than are men who don't exercise. Still just want to sit there and watch *Dancing with the Stars*?

7. Exercise is fun: Exercise and physical activity can be a fun way to spend some time. It gives you a chance to unwind, enjoy the outdoors or simply engage in activities that make you happy. Physical activity can also help you connect with family or friends in a fun social setting. Take a dance class, hit the hiking trails, join a soccer team, make a fitness pact with your best friend. Find a physical activity you enjoy, and just do it. If you get bored, try something new.

Truly, there is something on that list of 7 benefits for EVERYONE!! So latch onto your reason and commit that exercise will be a part of your life from here on out. Today is the first day of the rest of your life – you have the opportunity to start over in this very moment. It doesn't matter if you can't walk to the end of your driveway without getting winded – make the decision to start right now, where you are with what you have. You are not in competition with anyone but yourself and BETTER is a great word. Strive for just a little bit better every time.

The *Release* Exercise Plan

In the *Release* Plan, we advocate exercising, ideally, 6 days per week, incorporating cardiovascular interval training (to elevate metabolism and burn fat) 3 days per week and strength training (to build muscle) 3 days per week. At *MyReleasePlan.com* you can find a whole variety of interval training and strength training workouts to choose from or to give you ideas so you can create your own. The fact is that there is no one PERFECT workout – no cookie cutter approach that will work for everyone – exercise is very individual and very personal. Plus, when you are committing to doing an activity 6 days per week, it must be something you enjoy or you will not stick with it and you will not see the desired results.

Here's a great example. Our daughter, Nicki, is 17 years old. She was a teeny-tiny wisp of a girl when she was younger (even her nickname was "Munchkin"), but as puberty ensued she started to gain weight. The extra weight really damaged Nicki's self-image. She felt as though she were some kind of freak or something. Her mom and sister were very thin – what had she done to deserve this punishment? Deb had always mandated that the girls participate in some extracurricular activity that required them to move. In light of the fact that nothing else struck her fancy, Nicki chose to learn karate along with Deb starting at 9 years old. She really enjoyed it at first, but as the years wore on she got bored. Then boredom turned into outright dread of karate nights. There was a period of time when she actually quit, but she started again shortly thereafter because she is stubborn like her mother, and she wanted her black belt when she turned 16. Although many people around her found karate to be a fantastic way to get in shape and release weight (like Angie), Nicki's mindset prevented her from reaping those same benefits, and although she "dieted" and exercised 6 days per week (she went to 3-4 karate classes per week, plus she biked and even tried weightlifting for a while), she just kept gaining weight. The day after Nicki's black belt test (which she passed with flying colors) we moved to Florida and Nicki quit karate (presumably forever). She researched different exercises and decided that she wanted to give yoga a try. For 6 months she went to 3-4 90-minute "hot" yoga classes per week (the kind where the room is like 105°F and incredibly humid) and did interval training workouts the other 2-3 days per week. She hated it and her weight kept creeping up, despite watching what she ate and all the exercise.

In October, 2011 Nicki approached Deb and asked for help – she needed an accountability partner to help her get her weight under control. She was scared and depressed and a bit desperate. So, they created a 30 day contract where Nicki would eat and exercise according to the *Release* Plan principles, plus she would journal her perfect life for 15 minutes every single day (a practice we call imagineering, which we'll explain very soon in the Spirit section). An appropriately motivating reward and consequence were agreed upon and an accountability agreement was signed. After 30 days there wasn't much of a physical change, but there was a noticeable improvement in her attitude. They agreed to continue the contract for another 30 days with a new reward/consequence – same deal: eat and exercise according to the *Release* Plan and written imagineering every single day. Nicki was still hating yoga and biking, and although she was hopelessly hooked on the imagineering, there was still little noticeable physical change.

The accountability contracts continued and in early March, Nicki presented a proposal. Her 6 month contract at the yoga studio was coming to an end and she wanted to stop yoga – she didn't like it and it wasn't working for her. She proposed that she start walking a 3-4 mile loop for an hour per day, 6 days per week. We consulted over this proposal and set some very stringent guidelines, but agreed to let Nicki choose her exercise. What happened next was nothing short of amazing. Nicki did indeed start walking 6 days per week and her imagineering continued (as I am writing this we are celebrating Nicki's 180th straight day of imagineering today – 6 MONTHS – an incredible accomplishment) and as if by magic the weight started falling off her body. Clothes that had been skin tight only the month before were suddenly loose. Deb and I would look at her and marvel at how quickly her transformation was progressing. But more importantly, Nicki started seeing the change as well and actually began to CRAVE exercise. She was actually eager to go for her walks. Something inside her had shifted – it was her BELIEF that she could actually do this – she wasn't a freak of nature who was destined to be fat. She saw the possibilities and then saw them manifesting in her physical body. Her entire self-image changed in just few months and with it, her entire attitude, demeanor and outlook on life. She has transformed from a moody, self-centered, depressed teenager into a hopeful, cheerful, helpful, completely pleasant person to be around. So, if *Release* can work for the most hormonal of teenage girls, there is absolutely no reason why it won't work for YOU! Remember, it was when she finally started following **ALL** aspects of the *Release* Plan that she finally saw results – eating, exercising (finding something she liked) and imagineering – mind, body and spirit!

Interval Training

Whether you are currently a competitive athlete or could "go for gold" in the Couch Potato Olympics, there are REAL benefits to be reaped by adding interval training to your fitness regimen. At its most basic level, interval training simply means varying the intensity of your workout session - alternating bursts of higher intensity exercise with low to moderate intensity intervals for the entire workout. For example, jog for one minute then sprint for twenty seconds and repeat this pattern for 10 minutes; or if you are just starting out, go for a walk and alternate walking at a regular pace with walking at a faster pace. We want to impress upon you that this is all about training to your own level – you should push yourself and strive for "better" each day, but killing yourself right out of the gate is not going to do anyone any good at all!

There are so many benefits to interval training and it really offers amazing results in so many areas. Have you ever started an exercise program – say running – and found that after a few weeks you weren't progressing? You decided, "I'm going to run for 45 minutes 3 days per week." And you did it. And you experienced some results, but then all of a sudden you stalled out – you stopped losing weight, or getting faster or going further, or whatever your measure of "better" was. Does that sound familiar? Interval training takes care of those performance plateaus forever!! Interval training keeps your body guessing – it's never the same old routine.

Interval training:

1. Burns more calories and fat. Two minutes of moderate-intensity exercise is about the same as one minute of vigorous exercise. By adding interval training, you'll burn more calories than if you exercised at a steady pace.
2. Increases aerobic fitness. You'll be able to exercise at a harder intensity for a longer period of time, which, in turn, translates to having more energy throughout the day for ALL of your activities!
3. Saves time. Because interval training burns more calories and fat, you won't have to work out as long to get your desired results.
4. Tackles boredom. By changing up your intervals you can rejuvenate a tired workout routine, which keeps you engaged and motivated.

Interval training is all about ramping your level of exertion up for short bursts of time so that your heart rate elevates and then back down again, over and over again. Interval training is hard work, but the effort is worth it. We would be hard pressed to think of another form of exercise that offers more "bang for your buck" – more benefit for the time required – than interval training. Plus, interval training gives you an added bonus in that you continue to burn calories at an elevated rate long after your workout is over! If you just head out for a jog and run at the same speed for, say, 30 minutes, you will indeed burn calories while you are running, but as soon as the workout is finished, the extra calorie burning is over. Conversely, with interval training, you will actually experience an "after burn effect" where you will actually continue to burn more calories for hours after your workout is complete.

Sample Interval Training Workouts
(find additional workouts at MyReleasePlan.com)

12-Minute Fat Blaster
We love this workout when we are in a time crunch because it is over in a jiffy, but you definitely know you have worked! You

can do this work out on a stationary bike, on a real bike, running, using an elliptical machine, etc. The key is to be able to get to your maximum intensity quickly, because the high-intensity intervals are fairly short. In this workout you will warm up, then move through 8 rounds of 20 seconds at your maximum exertion level (Intensity Index (II) = 10), then 1 minute at an moderate exertion level (Intensity Index (II) = 6), ending with a cool down.

Warm up for 2 minutes (II = 6)
Hi-intensity interval – 20 seconds (II = 10)
Recovery interval – 60 seconds (II = 6)
Hi-intensity interval – 20 seconds (II = 10)
Recovery interval – 60 seconds (II = 6)
Hi-intensity interval – 20 seconds (II = 10)
Recovery interval – 60 seconds (II = 6)
Hi-intensity interval – 20 seconds (II = 10)
Recovery interval – 60 seconds (II = 6)
Hi-intensity interval – 20 seconds (II = 10)
Recovery interval – 60 seconds (II = 6)
Hi-intensity interval – 20 seconds (II = 10)
Recovery interval – 60 seconds (II = 6)
Hi-intensity interval – 20 seconds (II = 10)
Recovery interval – 60 seconds (II = 6)
Hi-intensity interval – 20 seconds (II = 10)
Recovery interval – 60 seconds (II = 6)
Cool Down – 2 minutes (II = 4)

20 Minute No-Excuses Workout

"I don't have time to exercise" will never be a valid excuse again with this quick and incredibly effective high-intensity interval training workout! This is a basic interval training workout that you can find on most electronic machines in a gym (elliptical machine, lifecycle, treadmill, stationary bicycle, stairclimber, etc.) – the trick is to adjust settings so that it really does take you to the appropriate intensity level during the workout, which may take some trial and error. But there is no need for fancy machines, just put on some sneakers and go for a walk, a jog or a run and keep track of time and your intensity index as follows:

Minute	Activity
1-2	Warm Up (II=5)
3	Walk/Jog/Run (II=6)
4	Walk/Jog/Run (II=7)
5	Walk/Jog/Run (II=8)
6	Walk/Jog/Run (II=9)
7	Walk/Jog/Run (II=6)
8	Walk/Jog/Run (II=7)
9	Walk/Jog/Run (II=8)
10	Walk/Jog/Run (II=9)
11	Walk/Jog/Run (II=6)
12	Walk/Jog/Run (II=7)
13	Walk/Jog/Run (II=8)
14	Walk/Jog/Run (II=9)
15	Walk/Jog/Run (II=6)
16	Walk/Jog/Run (II=7)
17	Walk/Jog/Run (II=8)
18	Walk/Jog/Run (II=9)
19	Walk/Jog/Run (II=10)
20	Cool Down (II=5)

For the cool down, walk, breathing in through your nose and out through your mouth until you are able to breathe normally and easily carry on a conversation.

To measure your level of exertion according to our Intensity Index numbers, use this as a guide:

II = 1 would be about the amount of exertion required to sit on the couch and watch TV;

II=5 allows you to easily carry on a conversation while engaging in the activity you are doing; and

II=10 is an all-out effort through which you would not be able to converse, breathe in through your nose and out through your mouth, or sustain for a long period of time.

We typically do interval training workouts three times per week and none of these workouts lasts longer than 20 minutes. They are quick, intense, and wickedly effective sessions, and the beautiful part is that interval training works for everyone, regardless of your current fitness level!

As your fitness improves, you will be able to:

- Exercise harder during the high intensity intervals. You started off doing a light jog, but now you may be able to sprint.
- Shorten the recovery interval. For instance, instead of running for 20 seconds and recovering for 60 seconds, perhaps your run for 30 seconds and recover for 50 seconds.
- Recover more quickly. As you get in better shape, you'll need less time to recover between high intensity intervals.

Adding speed to your workout is just one way to interval train. You could also:

- Add incline. If you are using a treadmill, you can adjust the incline during your high-intensity intervals, or exercise on a hilly terrain outdoors.
- Add resistance. If you are using a stationary bike or elliptical trainer, turn up the resistance a few notches to add intensity to your workout.

If you have never really exercised or if it's been years since you did more than walk to the mailbox or from the car to the office, start with walking - you'll be building muscles in your legs and you'll be getting a cardio workout to boot. As your fitness level improves you will be able to go farther and do more.

We think it goes without saying, but let's say it anyway, if you are just starting an exercise program of any kind, do yourself a favor and stop by your doctor's office for a checkup.

Tell him/her what you are planning to do and get their medical stamp of approval. But don't let that become an excuse for stalling – just get up and go for a walk for 30 minutes, 3 times per week until your doctor can see you. Then, introduce the interval training.

Once you have the concept of interval training down you will find that you can easily design your own workouts to accommodate your schedule, based on the activities you like to do. We have compiled a whole assortment of interval training workout options for you at *MyReleasePlan.com* – boredom need never be a problem – EVER again.

Strength Training

We believe that strength training should be a part of any fitness plan, but we know that no matter how many different ways we say it, some of you just will NOT lift weights and that's fine. Strength training on the *Release* Plan does not mean rushing out and buying a bunch of equipment or joining an expensive gym – there are plenty of strength training exercises that you can do with no special equipment at all – just your body weight. Many people have an incorrect perception about strength training. We are not talking about "bodybuilding," per se. Strength training is about improving muscle strength and muscle tone. For men, who have naturally higher levels of testosterone, it usually does mean an increase in muscle size; however, women tend to increase the tone without significantly increasing the muscle size. It is just not possible for a woman to look like those ladies in the muscle magazines without taking a whole host of supplements that are specifically designed to increase bulk – and that is certainly NOT what the *Release* Plan is about. In reality, most women who really try to "bulk up" through weightlifting can't do it. Our version of strength training has nothing to do with a bunch of Incredible Hulk wannabes "pumping iron" in a gym. Rather, it is about capitalizing on the incredible benefits that come from adding strength training to your overall fitness plan.

There are as many different approaches to strength training as there are experts in the field. We, your authors, lift weights three times per week alternating focus on upper body muscle groups during one session and lower body muscle groups the next – each of our weightlifting workouts is an hour long (because there are two of us sharing the equipment – when only one of us works out, the time required is between 30-45 minutes). In our martial arts training we do a variety of strength training exercises that are incredibly effective, but only require manipulating our own body weight in different ways; no equipment, weights, machines, etc. needed. Our goal in this section of the book is to open your eyes to the benefits of strength training and to expand your awareness and change your perspective so you can do some research and some experimentation and find what works for you. We have also compiled a library of strength training exercises and workouts, with and without weights, at *MyReleasePlan.com*.

1. The most obvious benefit of strength training is that you will add definition to your muscles and have a more fit and toned body, regardless if you are a man or a woman. If you want your body to look toned and defined once the extra fat has been released, then strength training is where that definition will come from.

2. Strength training protects bone health and muscle mass. Shockingly, after puberty, whether you are a man or a woman, you begin to lose about 1 percent of your bone and muscle strength every year. Strength training is one of the best ways to halt, prevent and even reverse bone and muscle loss! As a matter of fact, Deb had tests that showed she had osteopenia and was well on her way to osteoporosis, but was able to reverse it completely through nutrition and strength training.

3. Strength training makes you stronger and fitter. Strength training is also called resistance training because it involves strengthening and toning your muscles by contracting them against a resisting force. There are two types of resistance training - both make you stronger and can get you into better shape:

    a. Isometric resistance, which involves contracting your muscles against a non-moving object, such as against the floor in a push-up.

b. Isotonic strength training, which involves contracting your muscles through a range of motion, such as when you lift and lower a dumbbell.

4. Strength training helps you develop better body mechanics. A by-product of strength training is that your balance, posture and coordination will improve. Strength training can reduce your risk of falling by as much as 40 percent, a huge benefit, especially as you get older.

5. Strength training plays a role in disease prevention and alleviating the debilitating symptoms of some maladies. For instance, strength training has proven to be as effective as medication in decreasing arthritis pain. It can help post-menopausal women increase their bone density and reduce the risk of bone fractures. Strength training, along with other healthy lifestyle changes, can also help improve glucose control, which is incredibly important for individuals who suffer from diabetes.

6. Strength training boosts energy levels and improves your mood by elevating your level of endorphins (natural opiates produced by the brain), which will make you feel great. Strength training has also been shown to be a great antidepressant, to help you sleep better, and to improve your overall quality of life. You see, pills just mask symptoms; whereas, strength training goes to the source of the problem and rectifies it. Think about it , a headache is a symptom that something is not right with your body – a headache is NOT a symptom of an aspirin deficiency!

7. Strength training translates to more calories burned. You certainly burn calories during strength training, but, just like with interval training, your body continues to burn calories long AFTER you finish your workout!!! In layman's terms it is called the "afterburn," which is simply the extra calories your body burns while it is recovering from intense exercise (restocking oxygen and glycogen in the muscles, reducing body temperature, repairing muscle fibers, etc.) More calories are used to make and maintain muscle than fat, and in fact strength training can boost your metabolism by as much as 15 percent. So yes, it absolutely IS possible to burn lots of calories while

you sit around doing nothing, but you have to EARN it first!!

Strength Training on the *Release* Plan

The first thing you need to realize is that strength training as we define it on the *Release* Plan is all about quality – not about quantity. It's about pushing yourself as far as you can go within a defined period of time, with the goal being to go just a little bit further or do one more rep or lift just a little bit more weight than you did before next time. People seem to think that more is better – that we should always be striving to workout longer, but that kind of logic is nonsensical to us. The goal is to not only get better as we go along but more efficient as well.

As we said before, please don't think that lifting weights, buying expensive machines, or investing in a gym membership is the only way to do strength training. Pushups, sit ups, tricep dips, pull ups, jump squats, lunges, and mountain climbers are all examples of exercises that provide strength training. Too many people put off adding strength training to their exercise regimen because they feel they have to wait until they can afford to purchase equipment or join a gym, but there are plenty of things you can do to get started without spending a penny. Don't let Mr. X win that argument, because it is totally invalid!!

Walking can be a wonderful example of strength training in the beginning!! Think about it, if you are new to exercise or if it has been a long while since you have been very physically active, you are starting from ground zero, and there is no better exercise in the beginning than walking – for interval workouts and for strength training. As you begin a walking program, you set a defined period of time – say 30 minutes – and just walk. The next time you walk, strive to go a bit further in the same 30 minutes, then a bit further and a bit further. Over time you can start swinging your arms for added resistance; you can carry light handheld weights; as you get even more advanced you can fill empty milk jugs with sand or dirt and carry them on your walk. Then perhaps you choose to add jogging and start the process all over again. There is always something more you can do to challenge yourself each and every day – to push YOU to YOUR personal best!

As you develop your strength training regimen it is critical that you change it up about every 4 weeks. You continue to work the same muscle groups, but you will change the exercise you use to work them. This is where *MyReleasePlan.com* can come in really handy! It can be a daunting task to come up with even ONE full workout, much less changing exercises each month! We have a whole library of exercises for you to pick and choose from! There are two main reasons for varying your strength training workouts over time:

The first reason is psychological – the same old same old gets BORING and you can actually start to dread your exercise sessions!! Changing your workout every so often keeps things new and interesting, so you are less likely to give in to Mr. X when he pops his head up and tells you it is okay to skip a day.

The second reason is physiologically based and is even more important. There is a training phenomenon that Canadian endocrinologist, Hans Selye, postulated and researched called General Adaptation Syndrome (GAS) that explains how the body responds to stress. This applies to the *Release* Plan because interval training and strength training subject the body to large amounts of stress. There are three distinct phases to GAS:

1. Alarm Reaction: In this first phase, the body immediately reacts to stress. This is why people generally experience noticeable results very quickly at the beginning of a fitness program. Since the body is not used to exercise, muscle growth is induced and strength increases rapidly due to intermuscular, intramuscular, and neural adaptations.
2. Resistance: In this phase, the body begins to adapt to the stress it is being subjected to after a period of time. The onset of the resistance phase is not the same from person to person, depending in large part to the amount of stress one's body is used to.
3. Exhaustion: In this phase, the body can no longer endure the

stress and overtraining sets in. This is why the *Release* Plan advocates a Free Week every 4 months or so where you eat what you want and you don't exercise.

By varying your strength training regimens (and your interval training workouts as well) you can avoid entering the Resistance Stage of GAS and keep progressing toward your goals! This is HUGE!!

If you want to start lifting weights, we have included a number of wonderful reference resources in the "Next Level" section as well as on *MyReleasePlan.com*. There are so many fantastic books and websites and such that already exist, it's just silly to try to reinvent the wheel!

We understand that it can be tempting to just put the exercise part "on the shelf" for now. Logic would tell you that modifying your diet and tackling the self-image piece should be good enough for a start. However, this is not a cafeteria plan – you can't pick one thing from column A and something from column B and leave column C untouched. The *Release* Plan is a holistic approach to achieving REAL and PERMANENT weight release by adopting a whole new lifestyle.

Think about it, there are lots of people out there who desire that elusive "6-pack" musculature in their abdominal region, but it is just not there. The truth is that it is not all that difficult to tone your abdominal region – look at Angie's "after" pictures in Chapter 13 – those abs were not visible on January 1st!! Here's the paradox: Releasing weigh without working out will never give you the results you seek. Sure, your weight will decrease and your pant size will go down, but without the muscle tone that exercise provides, all that extra skin will just hang on your body, which is never attractive. That's why you can go to the beach and see a very thin woman or man in a bathing suit, but they look flabby even though they are obviously very lean. It's a flabby, wasted look, not a fit, healthy look.

On the other hand, If you exercise without releasing the extra weight on your body, you may have beautiful muscles, but no one will ever see them because they are covered up by a thick blanket of fat – so that doesn't work either! When you combine the right mindset, with the right nutritional program AND then right exercise plan you create a beautiful physique that is lean, strong and healthy. Remember, SKINNY people may look good in clothes, but FIT people look good naked!!

OUCH!! Why am I so sore?

You made the decision to start the *Release* Plan and you did a walk/run interval workout 2 days ago and a circuit of strength training exercises yesterday. This morning you woke up and could barely get out of bed. What's wrong? Have you injured yourself? Not likely. You are experiencing delayed onset muscle soreness (DOMS) which describes the muscle pain, muscle soreness or muscle stiffness that occurs in the day or two after exercise. This muscle soreness is most frequently felt when you begin a new exercise program, change your exercise routine, or dramatically increase the duration or intensity of your exercise routine. Although it can be alarming for new exercisers, delayed onset muscle soreness is a normal response to unusual exertion and is part of an adaptation process that leads to greater stamina and strength as the muscles recover and build (remember the Alarm Reaction phase in the General Adaptation Syndrome we covered earlier?). This sort of muscle pain is not the same as the muscle pain or fatigue you experience during exercise, which is caused by a build up of lactic acid in your muscles. Delayed soreness is also unlike the acute, sudden and sharp pain of an injury such as a muscle strain or sprain that occurs during activity and often causes swelling or bruising (if you experience an acute, jabbing pain, you should cease exercise and see your doctor to make sure there are no serious injuries). The delayed muscle soreness of DOMS is generally at its worst within the first 2 days following a new, intense activity and slowly subsides over the next few days.

Delayed onset muscle soreness is thought to be a result of microscopic tearing of the muscle fibers. The amount of tearing (and soreness) depends on how hard and how long you exercise and what type of exercise you do. Any movement you aren't used to can lead to DOMS, but eccentric muscle contractions (movements that cause the muscle to forcefully contract while it lengthens – for example, running down stairs, running downhill, lowering weights and the downward motion of squats and push-ups) seem to cause the most soreness. In addition to small muscle tears there can be associated swelling in a muscle which may contribute to soreness. So at its most basic level, when you exercise you tear down muscle fibers and the soreness you feel is a result of your body's immune response rebuilding the muscles (more defined and stronger each time). The peak of the soreness will be at around 24-36 hours post-exercise. The good news is that it doesn't last very long!

There are some things you can do to help prevent or alleviate DOMS:

1. Eat some high quality protein (chicken, cottage cheese, a protein shake, etc.) as soon after exercise as possible. Muscles are comprised of protein; you will be feeding your body what it requires to repair itself.
2. As unappealing as it may sound, one of the best ways to help reduce the duration of the soreness is to do more of the exercise that made you sore in the first place. If your chest and arms are sore from push-ups, do 2 or 3 slow push-ups from your knees or against a wall. If your thighs are screaming at you from the sets of squats you did, just do a few nice slow, easy squats. If your soreness is the result of a run, go for a short walk.

Unfortunately, some level of soreness when you start a new exercise regimen or when you change up your fitness routine is normal and natural and even desirable – discomfort indicates growth in all areas of your life! Here's the good news! Your body, as you have read, is amazingly adaptable and the intensity of the soreness you experience will diminish with each repetition of the workout. For example, if you start a new strength training routine on Monday, you may find that by Tuesday evening you are scarcely able to move the areas of your body that you focused on during your workout. You may wonder how on earth you will be able to repeat the workout again on Friday! However, by Friday, the soreness has lessened enough for you to do it all over again.

Then on Saturday night you notice that you are not nearly as sore after Friday's workout as you were after Monday's – and so it goes. With each passing workout your body will adapt a bit more and a bit more, which is another reason why you want to change your routine every 4 weeks or so.

The *Release* Nutrition and Exercise Plan Summary

- Eat five to six, small meals per day, depending on the number of waking hours in your day, spaced ~2-3 hours apart
- Each meal should consist of roughly equal amounts of protein and carbohydrate (for the average woman 20 grams at each meal is ideal), but don't make yourself crazy about it - just follow the "fist/palm" guidelines
- Add vegetables to at least two meals per day
- Incorporate meal and protein shakes into your daily plan for inexpensive, convenient, quick to prepare meals
- Consume protein before bedtime to facilitate your body's repair and regeneration during the night
- Plan your meals each week – don't leave your nutrition to chance!
- Drink at least 6 **16 oz.** glasses of water per day
- Every 7th day, throw all the rules out the window and eat whatever you wish.
- Every 4 months or so, take a break for a week – eat what you want and take a break from structured exercise as well
- Exercise 6 days per week – 3 days of interval training and 3 days of strength training
- Find a strength training program that works for you – if you are a beginner, start with walking and go from there – JUST START! Join us at *MyReleasePlan.com* for lots of great workout ideas!
- Strive for continual improvement in your workouts – a little further, a little more intensity – within a defined period of time. Remember, it's about quality, not quantity! Go for YOUR personal best each workout.

Deb Cheslow & Angie Flynn

Spirit

"Love and desire are the spirit's wings to great deeds."
–Johann Wolfgang von Goethe

Deb Cheslow & Angie Flynn

CHAPTER THIRTEEN

Spirit Is Perfect

We believe very strongly that true, lasting, meaningful change in any area of our lives requires the mind, the body and the spirit working in concert. We have covered, although only on a surface level, the concept of Mind and self-image and how you must change your self-image to be in alignment with your goals or you will never be able to sustain the behavior required to get, and keep, you there. We have covered the actions that need to be taken by the body in terms of proper nutrition and exercise and the details of the *Release* program in practice. Now we need to talk about Spirit, because it is probably the most neglected aspect of the "mind-body-spirit connection" and yet it is critical that you have an awareness of it because spirit is the glue that binds all the rest together.

One note: This section of the book is NOT about religion. We're not going there. Whether you are devoutly religious or an atheist, we believe our philosophy of Spirit will be congruent with your beliefs.

All science and all religion teach that we have unlimited potential locked within us and that we are capable of incredible feats. Our spiritual DNA is perfect – at our core, we are absolutely perfect beings. When we speak of spirit, we are referring to it as the amorphous but ever-present, infinite substance or energy present individually in all living things, which develops and grows as an integral aspect of a living being. Although human beings are flawed, spirit is PERFECT!

Deb Cheslow & Angie Flynn

CHAPTER FOURTEEN

Your Higher Self

As human beings we live on three planes of existence simultaneously – we are innately spiritual beings, we are gifted with an intellect and we reside in a physical body. The intellect is the medium through which our spiritual self and our physical self communicate. As purely spiritual beings we do not have any of the limitations that our physicality imposes on us – spirit does not catch a cold, it does not break bones, it does not get stressed out and it certainly doesn't raid the refrigerator at midnight!! Our spiritual self is infinite in its capacity and its capability and that infinite possibility is screaming to be expressed. That's what is happening when we get the urge to do something new – a true DESIRE to go beyond what we have experienced in our physical life to date. That urge – that desire – is our spiritual side communicating with our physical self through our intellect. Our intellect creates thoughts and images of all this cool stuff spirit wants us to physically DO. Unfortunately, more times than not, all the virus code that has infected our subconscious mind (the negative paradigms) squashes the idea as soon as we start to get excited about it.

Think about it for a second, what would your life be if every time you thought "I should do Y" (whatever "Y" is), you actually DID it? Because each time you think "I should…" it's a message coming from your perfect spiritual self, urging you on to live a more expansive, fuller life. When you think of it in those terms, isn't it EXCITING? Doesn't it take just a little bit of the fear and the unknown out of the equation? You will NEVER be driven or have a desire to do something you are incapable of achieving. It doesn't work that way.

Everything that has manifested on the physical plane has spirit as its ultimate source – it existed on the spiritual plane before someone got the great idea to "invent" it and took the actions necessary to bring it into physical reality. Think about the Wright brothers and the airplane or Thomas Edison and the light bulb; or Edmund Hilary and his unrelenting, burning desire to reach the summit of Mount Everest, even though everyone who had attempted it before had failed or died trying. Things we consider commonplace, like the computer or the smartphone or the microwave oven, are all the products of someone's unreasonable fantasy.

What does this have to do with you achieving your ideal body? Great question! The answer... EVERYTHING!! We have discussed self image and how you will never outperform what you believe yourself to be. Each of us has spiritual perfection locked inside of us, but we have covered it up with so much junk – the habits and conditioning – that we can't even recognize it. If each of us stripped away all of the junk that is cluttering our subconscious mind, we would all have the exact same self-image – an image of pure, spiritual perfection. Can you ever get there? Probably not. But you CAN do exactly what all those famous inventors throughout history did – they became obsessed with an unreasonable fantasy. They tapped into spirit, which is absolutely infinite, and created an image of what they wanted in their minds and they focused and took action on it day in and day out. They allowed themselves to be inundated by their goal on all three planes of their existence.

Techniques for Tuning into Spirit

Imagineering

Imagineering is a combination of the words "imagination" and "engineering." The term was coined by Alcoa in the 1940's, but is more popularly associated with Walt Disney. The idea behind imagineering is to take the limits off your thoughts about what is possible and to let your imagination go where logic says it cannot – to allow yourself to dream again like you did when you were a child.

You can use the concept of imagineering in any area of your life that you want to improve, but in the context of your *Release* program, we want you to spend 30 minutes imagineering your end result – your ideal body - each day – 15 minutes of written imagineering and then 15 minutes spent just thinking about what you wrote and FEELING it. Let go of logic and circumstantial restraints and WRITE! No one is going to read it but you – it's an absolutely private exchange between you and the universe. No one is checking your spelling, grammar or punctuation, so let it flow. It can be difficult in the beginning – we get so used to being "logical" and "rational" that taking the lid off and dreaming BIG can be really hard!!

Angie's Story: I remember the first time I tried imagineering – I felt so self-conscious, even though I was the only one who was ever going to read what I wrote. The first time I wrote that I wanted a brand new, custom-built BMW X5 SAV or that I wanted "6-pack abs," I think I actually blushed with embarrassment of such audacious wishes!! But you know what? That BMW is sitting in my garage right now – it's MINE!! And, those 6-pack abs are very real – I created them! If I had not dared to dream I could have them, I would probably still be driving my twelve year old Chrysler minivan and would still be busting out of my size 12 jeans!

So, DREAM BIG!!! Start each imagineering session with "I am so happy and grateful now that…" and let the details of your ideal body pour out onto the paper as if it is already a fact in your life right now. Look back at what you wrote in the Mind section to get you started. Don't worry about HOW it will happen – that's not your concern at this point. The most important part is to only give energy to what you WANT – give no thought to what you don't want (for instance, write "I am so happy and grateful now that I am at my ideal weight of 130 lbs" rather than "I am so happy and grateful now that I am not fat anymore"). The subconscious mind only processes images; it doesn't hear verbs, adverbs, qualifiers, etc. If you think "not fat anymore" your subconscious mind only processes "fat" and has a very clear image of a fat person – YOU! Remember, we think in pictures!! So, what do you think you'll be attracting into your life? That's right, FAT!

Deb Cheslow & Angie Flynn

We have a client who has been doing amazing things in her professional life, but has been struggling in her personal life, especially with her weight. We were talking to her about what her stumbling block was (as she is an incredible practitioner of this material) and she said, "I just don't know. I have pictures all over my kitchen and my office of what I want to look like and reminders to eat healthy. For instance, on my refrigerator I have picture of a cheeseburger, a milkshake and a big, fat butt and then a picture of a salad, a glass of water and a headless photo of a slim woman in a bikini." We immediately and practically simultaneously said "Get rid of the picture of the fat butt." She argued that she needed it there to remind her of what would happen if she kept eating out of control. Deb asked her which picture had the greater impact on an emotional level – the fat butt or the bikini picture. She admitted that the fat butt picture literally made her cringe every time she saw it. Deb then explained how the emotional response to the fat picture would keep her gaining weight forever because her subconscious mind was processing "fat butt, fat butt, fat butt" every time she set foot inside her kitchen. We could see the "a-ha" moment in her eyes as she realized that she was sabotaging herself with the images she was inundating her subconscious mind with.

Now, imagine that you have already achieved your goal. Detail in writing how you FEEL now that you have achieved what you want – become emotionally involved in your vision. THAT'S how you change the paradigms and your self-image – by getting emotionally involved with the IMAGES associated with what you want.

Again, we know that some people have difficulty with the concept of imagineering in the beginning. They know they want a change, but it's been so long since they allowed themselves to dream beyond the here and now that they have trouble getting started. Just begin *"I am so happy and grateful now that..."* and then take some piece of the life that will manifest when you attain your goal, and then write about that small piece. Just start writing about SOMETHING. Over time the words will begin to flow from your mind onto the paper and intuition will lead you to envision things you want to be, do, or have in other areas of your life. Soon there will be no stopping you – you'll be a dream machine!!

One important note – we have tested this process over and over again and we can tell you that typing on a keyboard is not the same as taking a pen and paper and kicking it old school. There is not the same mind-body connection when you are typing into a word processing document as there is when you are writing with a pen and paper. Actual writing on a sheet of paper causes your mind to think, thinking evokes images, those images cause feelings in your subconscious mind, the feelings move you into action and the action causes a re-action (a result). Then you can analyze your result, see if it is in line with what you want and then make adjustments in your imagineering to start the process all over again. The people we have worked with (including ourselves) who have tried it both ways (computer and pen/paper) have achieved significantly better and faster results with good old pen and paper. Another reason for the disparity in results between typing into a computer and writing by hand has to do with the level of brain activation achieved by each. In extremely simplistic terms, typing on a keyboard activates only eight neural pathways, while writing long-hand, regardless of the language you are writing in, activates over 10,000 neural pathways – you literally feel the thought when you write long hand!

Similarly, just *thinking* about what you want isn't good enough either because you can't control your logic when you just think about something. There will constantly be interruptions as logic wants to know, "Well how on earth are you going to do that?" The HOW is not important right now, just that you want it, and writing allows you to circumvent logic!

Let's look at some examples of good and bad imagineering:

Good

I am so happy and grateful now that I have reached my ideal weight. I love the way my body looks, feels and performs. It is a true pleasure to walk into my closet and choose what to wear each day, knowing that every piece fits me perfectly! I love the admiring looks I get from my husband/wife, realizing that they are so proud of what I have accomplished. I crave nutritious food and vigorous exercise and know that with each day I am creating a better, healthier, more vibrant body. I love my body and care for it in all ways...

Bad

I am so happy and grateful now that I have lost all the weight I was carrying around on my body. All the fat rolls are gone and I can actually touch my toes again. It feels so good now that my thighs don't rub together any longer when I walk and I can actually walk up a flight of stairs without getting out of breath. I actually threw away all of my fat clothes last week. I am so happy that people don't make rude comments about how fat I am anymore...

Can you see the difference between these two paragraphs? The first example relates life in all positive terms, while the second example is filled with imagery of what used to be – the fat rolls, the rude comments, the chafing thighs, the huffing and puffing up the stairs. The subconscious mind processes images, so it doesn't realize that you are talking about what used to be or what you are so glad is gone – it processes what you write – fat, fat rolls, fat clothes, nasty comments, etc. – and will do everything possible to make sure you get more of those things!!

Imagineering is a process - and it can be pretty darned frustrating at times. It's not like you just start writing one day and you wake up the next day at your ideal weight. It's an evolution. Changing the conditioning that's been with you for decades is HARD WORK!! And the more junk that's been heaped on you over those decades, the harder it is. But there is NOTHING better than when you wake up one day and realize that you really HAVE changed and that life IS better and you really DO need a telescope to see how far you've come.

IMAGINEERING: Summing it up

IMAGINEER **EVERY** DAY!

* Buy a cool notebook or binder and a nice pen that is dedicated just for your imagineering – make this time special for YOU;

- Enjoy 15 minutes of freeflow writing and then 15 minutes visualizing what you wrote in a relaxed state;
- Start with "I am so happy and grateful now that....."
- Describe your ideal body, health, fitness level, nutritional choices, exercise plan – whatever you feel like writing about that day - in the present tense as if it were already a fact;
- Only discuss what you want; do not give ANY energy to what you don't want.

This is one of those places where it is probably a good idea to remind you that you need to do exactly what we tell you if you want major results. Imagineering is one of those things where it is easy to put it off or let it go by the wayside when time is tight. Make imagineering a priority – better yet, make it a HABIT!! Habitualizing an action takes approximately 30 days (remember the discussion of the NASA experiment back in Chapter Five?). Hard schedule 15 minutes of writing time into your calendar if you have to, but don't just make a half-hearted commitment here. Imagineering is the single most effective way to change your self-image, but you have to do it every, single day! There have been days when we stagger into the house after a non-stop 15 hour day and all we want to do is fall into bed, but we still take those 15 minutes and imagineer – after all these years, we still do it EVERY SINGLE DAY!!

Listen to your vision

Take the description you wrote in the "Where Are You Going" section earlier in this book and actually record yourself reading it aloud using the voice recorder on your phone or a digital voice recorder. Then listen to it first thing in the morning (as soon as your eyes open reach for your recorder and listen to it) and last thing before you fall asleep at night. Listening to your vision is incredibly powerful – especially when it is you talking to YOU about the details. You are stimulating yet another one of your physical senses and the repetition of the images that are evoked when you listen to your recording are driving deep into your subconscious mind and are altering your self-image bit by bit.

When you make your recording make sure that your voice is up-beat, enthusiastic and animated – even to the point of over doing it. That enthusiasm will translate as you listen to the recording and you won't be able to help but get excited yourself. Conversely, if you just read your description of your ideal life in a monotone, ho-hum voice, you won't be excited at all – in fact, you are likely to depress yourself and start "logic"-ing yourself to death as you listen. So, get excited, enthusiastic and exuberant about your vision!!

Inundate Yourself with Your Goal

When you are imagineering on a daily basis and you have a vision of what you REALLY want, you need to help the image of that vision permeate your subconscious mind. You now know that you think in pictures and the purpose of imagineering is to create the *picture* of what you want in your life. The purpose of the repetition is to drive that image into your subconscious mind over and over and over again. The subconscious mind does not have the ability to choose what it accepts, so whatever you turn over to it repetitiously will be accepted as reality. The dissonance between your actual physical reality and what your subconscious PERCEIVES to be reality will cause you to act in ways that will manifest the perceived reality.

The best way we have found to generate the required level of repetition is to literally inundate yourself with your goal. Here are some examples of how to do that:

1. Imagineering: Writing is the BEST way to drive images into your subconscious mind. Writing causes thinking, thinking creates images, images stir the emotions, the emotional response drives the body into action and that action creates a result. You can then look at the new result and fine tune your imagineering until the results you are getting match what you want.

2. Carry a Goal Card: A goal card is simply a small card (like a business card) that you write your goal on and then carry with you in your pocket or purse. On it you write "I am so

happy and grateful now that…" and then write something that you REALLY want. You don't have to have any clue how you are you are going to get it; you just have to WANT it. Read it as often as possible. It is the repetition of the ideas that changes your thinking by allowing you to take your mind off your present circumstances and focusing it on what you want. An example could be: "I am so happy and grateful now I have reached my ideal weight of 138 lbs. I wear a size 4/6 and love the way my body looks, feels and performs. I am strong, healthy, and unstoppable." Goal cards work in any area of your life!! (You can download a complimentary goal card from our website at *MyReleasePlan.com*).

3. Use Affirmations: Affirmations are positive statements that describe a desired situation, and which are repeated many times, in order to impress the subconscious mind and trigger it into positive action. Like your goal statement, we suggest you start your affirmations with "I am so happy and grateful now that…" In order to ensure the effectiveness of the affirmations, they have to be repeated with attention, conviction, interest and desire. We suggest that you carry your affirmation statements around with your goal card and read them often! You can develop affirmation statements for any area of your life you wish to improve. Here are a couple of examples:
    a. I am so happy and grateful now that my mind, body and spirit are strong."
    b. I am so happy and grateful now that I always make healthy choices and only fuel my body with the highest quality food."
    c. "I am so happy and grateful now that I always have time for the people and things that are important to me."
4. Physically inundate your senses with your goal: Your instinctive response is to act on physical stimuli. In general, your perception of reality is based on what you take in from the outside world through your five senses. When you immerse your senses in what you want your life to be, it drives those images into your subconscious mind where they can move into form through your actions. Some examples of how to inundate your senses:

a.   Place pictures or post-it-notes on your mirror. Find a picture on the internet or in a magazine of someone with the body that you would love to have.

b.   Create vision boards (collections of pictures and words that show what you want – Pinterest.com is an excellent place to find all kinds of images for your board – a totally visual, image driven site).

c.   Use your goal card. Read it, touch it, say it out loud as often as possible.

d.   "Photoshop" your head onto a picture of the body you want.

e.   Rig your scale to always show your ideal weight! Go to *MyReleasePlan.com* and create an image of your perfect weight in a red, digital font. Print the image and tape it over your scale's display. Now every time you get on the scale you will look down and see yourself already at your ideal weight.

As we discussed earlier in this section, we live on three planes of existence simultaneously. Everything already exists on the spiritual plane and as soon as you think of something it exists on the intellectual plane. Think about that for a second, once you conceive an idea, you already possess it on two of the three planes of existence. By tapping into your higher, spiritual self you facilitate the manifestation of what you desire on the physical plane. Napoleon Hill said it very well, "We become what we think about most of the time." What you give energy to grows. If you want to reach your ideal weight you have to have thoughts of you at your perfect weight most of the time. The more you hold the image of what you want on the screen of your mind, the faster that image will be manifested on the physical plane. And the really cool part is that these techniques can work for anything in your life: your weight, your financial condition, your relationships, your career – ANYTHING!! All the concepts in this program are the same, it's just the application that changes!

CHAPTER FIFTEEN

Results

You are probably wondering how the first 90 days of the *Release* Plan worked for us. Okay, here it comes: Pictures, scale results, the whole she-bang!

Angie's Results

I had a tough time in January – I was technically following the plan, but I know that many of my portions were too big and I was still fudging on my water intake. I also wanted to give a week-by-week accounting of my weight, so I was getting on the scales every Saturday morning. That stupid number on the scales each week would either make or break my vibration for the whole day! As expected, I experienced a fairly easy, quick release of weight initially, but then I stalled out. Each week I would get on the scale and I would either be the same or even up a pound from the previous week and I would get so upset and frustrated, because I thought I was really working the plan.

On February 4th I came back from my weigh in angry. I told Deb that it wasn't working. She suggested that I stop getting on the scale, or if I wanted to put the results in the book, I should let her see the number, but not look myself. That's what we did. I let Deb record my weight and, although it killed me from a curiosity perspective, I had no idea what I weighed. I stepped up my imagineering and really focused on what I wanted my body to look like and how I wanted to feel and the clothes I wanted to wear. I especially focused on my abs because I really wanted one of those "6-packs." And I got on the scales repeatedly throughout the week and every time I looked down I saw my perfect weight staring back at me, thanks to the scale rigging technique discussed in the last chapter.

Within a couple of weeks my clothes started feeling looser. I could see the muscles in my arms, abs and legs becoming more and more visible and defined. Each week I made more progress and looked better. I no longer winced every time I looked in the mirror – I was proud of what I saw reflected back at me. I dropped 2 full dress sizes from a tight size 10 to a loose size 8. All that happened between February 4th and April 6th.

On April 6th we took "After" pictures. Anyone who has known me for more than 5 minutes knows that it took every ounce of courage I have to put on a bikini and let someone photograph me for a BOOK! After the shoot we had our final weigh in and I got to look this time. At first I was upset by what I saw – 152 pounds. After all that I had only lost 6 pounds – it didn't work? But then it dawned on me – that stupid scale was dictating my self-image. It was putting a mental ceiling on what I believed I was capable of achieving. In 2 months I had absolutely *transformed* my body – whether the scale showed that or not, I could look in the mirror and SEE the results! Of course, there are any number of reasons why the scale didn't tell the whole story – added muscle, water retention, the time of day, time of the month. The fact is that when I threw the scale away, it freed my mind to create the image of what I saw in my mind, unconstrained by my self-imposed limitations. If I can do it, YOU can do it!!

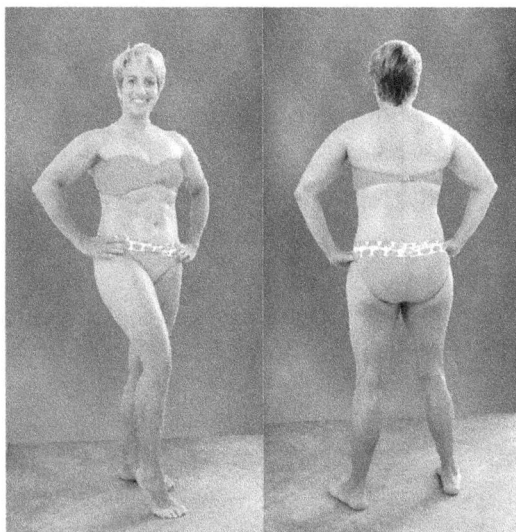

April 6, 2012 (after 90 days)

Angie Flynn

Age: 46
Start Weight: 158
End Weight: 152

Height: 5'5 ½"
Start size: 10/12
End size: 6/8

Deb's Results

I have been following the "Body" part of the *Release* Plan for over a decade and instinctively following the "Mind" and "Spirit" sections, so I didn't really expect amazing, transformational results physically. However, this was the first time I really used material presented in the "Mind" and "Spirit" sections and applied on a conscious level. Like Angie, I started the program by checking my weight progress each Saturday. Also like Angie, I found that after a couple of weeks, my weight plateaued and wouldn't budge!

I found my thoughts wandering from time to time to things about my body that I didn't like, which is absolutely the wrong thing to do, but I was frustrated by my lack of progress. In February it was apparent that Angie was having the same difficulties, so I suggested that we stop looking at the scale.

Once we took that silly scale out of the equation, incredible things began to happen. Even though I changed nothing else, my pants (which I bought in December and had professionally tailored to fit me perfectly), were suddenly getting looser. When I looked in the mirror, I saw new lines of definition in my arms and abs. My stomach was flatter than at any time since the birth of my daughters. By the end of March, every pair of pants I owned was gaping at the waist – to the point of needing to be altered again.

When I stepped on the scales on April 6th for our "After" weigh in, I found that I had lost 2 whole pounds. Many people might be upset by that, but I was more enthusiastic than ever, because I had finally found the answer; it was suddenly crystal clear to me that watching the scales each week was causing my stall. Once I began focusing on what I loved about my body and what I wanted it to look like, I got more of it. It all begins and ends with belief!!

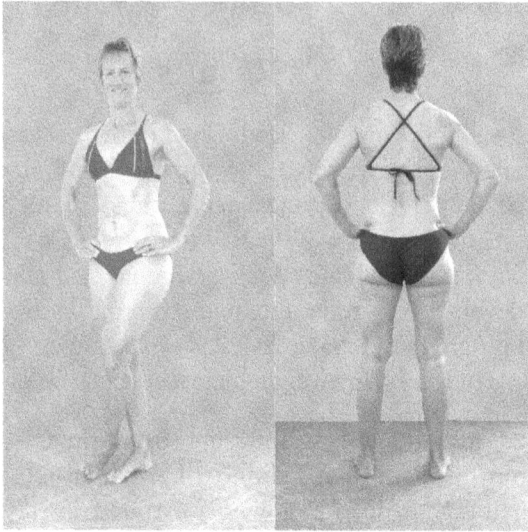

April 6, 2012 - after 12 YEARS!

Deb Cheslow

Age: 47	Height: 5'6"
Start Weight: 144	Start size: 8
End Weight: 142	End size: 6

At the end of the day, as countless people have proven, changing your self-image is so much more powerful than seeing a big drop on the scale. It is so freeing to no longer be ruled by a STUPID number on a STUPID scale, and let's face it, it's ridiculous to have your self-worth determined by a STUPID number!! When you change your self-image, the results you see on your body become permanent, which is why the *Release* Plan is so different from all other weight control programs! Here are the main keys to success:

1. THROW THE SCALE AWAY!!! If you can't bear to part with your precious scale, then rig it so it always shows your perfect weight.

2. This is a LIFESTYLE, not another "diet!" Deb has lived this way for 12 YEARS and her results speak for themselves. The *Release* Plan is about abundance and flexibility and enjoying your life, not about living in a bubble and enduring.

3. Self-image is absolutely KEY!! You must focus on what you want and give absolutely no energy to what you don't want. It doesn't matter if your love handles have love handles – you have to keep your focus on the body you want to be reflected back at you in the mirror! Use imagineering every day to help facilitate this process. And, for Heaven's sake, DO NOT allow the value you place on yourself to be dictated by a number spit out by a stupid mechanical device- the scale!

Deb Cheslow & Angie Flynn

The Next Level

"We are what we repeatedly do. Excellence, then, is not an act, but habit."
–Aristotle

Deb Cheslow & Angie Flynn

CHAPTER SIXTEEN

Kicking it Up a Notch

So that's the *Release* Plan – combining the right mindset and self-image with the right nutrition and fitness program so that your body releases the extra weight that it has been holding on to. If you do nothing more than what is prescribed in the first three sections of this book, you will achieve phenomenal results. But, many people, once they start altering their self-image and eating right and exercising, find that they feel so much better that they want to go even further. That's what The Next Level section is all about – suggesting some additional things for you to consider implementing in your life so you can feel even better and perform at even higher levels.

Deb Cheslow & Angie Flynn

CHAPTER SEVENTEEN

Next Level Nutrition

Now that you are fueling your body at the proper intervals with meals that are in the right amounts and the right combination of protein, fat and carbohydrate, there are some simple adjustments you can make to take it to the next level.

Buy Organic

You can buy almost any food, including candy, coffee and wine in an "organic" variety at just about any food store across the country. But is the health "bang" you get worth the extra "bucks" you have to spend? In our opinion, there are three main areas where we insist on organic products:

- Eggs: Eggs are a terrific source of protein, but factory farmed chickens are raised using a range of antibiotics and hormones to promote "health" of the animal and growth. Hormones in the eggs = hormones in your body! Organic eggs come from chickens that are raised on organic feed and are not given hormones or antibiotics (except in the case of an infectious outbreak). Organic eggs also have higher levels of vitamin E, omega-3 essential fatty acids and antioxidants.
- Milk: Some studies on supplements like recombinant bovine growth hormone (rBGH) used in conventional milk production have suggested links to early puberty and other hormonal abnormalities. Danish studies have shown that not only does organic milk have less of the bad stuff, but it also has more of the good stuff. Like organic eggs, organic milk has higher levels of vitamin E, omega-3 essential fatty acids and antioxidants.
- Meat: Animals (cows, chickens, fish, etc.) that are raised organically are not allowed to be fed antibiotics, bovine human growth hormone (rBGH), or other artificial drugs. Animals are also not allowed to eat genetically modified foods. Organically raised animals have been shown to be

significantly healthier than their factory-raised counterparts. We go back to the maxim "Garbage in, garbage out." Plus, in our experience, organic meat, poultry and fish are just so much tastier! Visit *MyReleasePlan.com* for links to locate an organic beef, poultry or fish supplier near you.

Supplementation

Unfortunately, even if every bite of food you put in your mouth is 100% organic, you are going to have a difficult time getting all the vitamins and minerals your body needs just from the food you eat. We live in a world where much of the soil used to raise crops is depleted of nutrients and where the water and air is polluted – it just is what it is.

The fact is that 99% of American adults fail to meet the USDA "Food Pyramid" dietary guidelines, according to an article reported in 1998 by the Council for Responsible Nutrition. The Anarem Report, which documents a government sponsored National Food Consumption Survey of over 21,500 individuals, showed that **not a single person** consumed 100% of the RDA for the following studied nutrients: protein, calcium, iron, vitamin A, vitamin C, thiamine, riboflavin, vitamin B-6, vitamin B-12, and magnesium. That is a scary statistic! And it gets even worse! Today's hectic, manic lifestyle makes it difficult to eat well. We eat on the run due to the fast-paced lives we lead. Very few families sit down to one good meal a day, let alone three. In single parent households and households in which both parents work it is common for healthy meals to be replaced by nutrient-poor fast foods in the name of convenience. The American Cancer Society and American Heart Association recommend that we consume 25-35 grams of fiber daily, but most people average only 7-14 grams a day. Our body's functions are so intertwined that one missing nutrient can affect the absorption and utilization of others, according to The Nutrition Almanac. In addition to that, studies show that most people experience stress every ten minutes during the day. Stress rapidly depletes B vitamins and vitamin C. These nutrients are critical to help us get the energy we need from our food and to keep our immune systems strong and healthy. Stress also causes muscles to contract, increasing our need for calcium and magnesium.

So, what do you do? The easy answer is to say take a daily multivitamin, but that raises a whole host of other issues! Almost all of the multivitamin brands that you can buy at the food store or the pharmacy are synthetic, chemically manufactured pills that travel the whole of your digestive tract and are eliminated into the toilet virtually untouched. They do your body little or no good at all. However, there are some brands of vitamins available that are processed differently so that they are bioavailable and actually nourish your cells and give your body what it needs to make up for the lack of nutrients in your diets. We recommend you find a good, bioavailable multivitamin/multimineral supplement and commit to taking it daily.

Angie's Story: My young son, Josh, had been plagued by allergies, asthma, colds, chronic coughing and the like for years. We practically lived at our pediatrician's office – the receptionist knew my voice immediately when I called for an appointment and we were on a first name basis with all of the office staff, nurses and technicians in the practice. We ate the "typical American diet" (translated, we ate like crap) and Josh took a children's chewable vitamin every day – that's what you are supposed to do, right? After I met Deb we were talking about Josh and she was asking me about the chronic cough he had suffered from for the past several months (it usually got worse during the exertion of his karate class). I told her I was at a loss; he had been on several courses of antibiotics, but the cough persisted. The next day she brought me a bottle of children's vitamins manufactured by a company she knew and trusted and suggested that I give them to Josh and see if they helped. I started him on the vitamins the next day. Within 48 hours Josh's cough was completely gone – not just better, but GONE! He had been hacking and coughing for nearly 6 months and it was gone! I didn't even think twice and ordered a supply of the vitamins for him. That was 2-1/2 years ago and Josh has been to the doctor once (for the flu) since then. He is the healthiest child I know. His allergies and asthma are completely gone.

Again, we cannot and will not promise medical miracles, but it is absolutely astonishing how much damage the human body can overcome when it is nourished in the proper way. Supplementation can be an excellent way to take your health to the next level by ensuring that you are getting adequate levels of the vitamins and minerals that you should be getting, but aren't, from the food you eat.

CHAPTER EIGHTEEN

Next Level Fitness

You have been following the *Release* Plan and have incorporated interval training and strength training into your fitness routine. You are feeling stronger than you have in a long time and are ready to take things to the next level.

MyReleasePlan.com

Join us at *MyReleasePlan.com* and experience the wide variety of interval training and strength training workouts for all fitness levels!

Sports Nutrition

We have integrated two specific products into our fitness program that have taken our workouts to the next level.

A Workout Maximizer Supplement: This is a protein shake formulation that is designed specifically for athletes. We find that we recover more quickly with less delayed onset muscle soreness using this product.

An Electrolite Replacement Sports Drink: People often make the mistake of thinking they will know when they need more fluids because they will feel thirsty. The fact is that by the time you notice thirst, you are already dehydrated and in a workout situation this can be a dangerous scenario! As you workout and perspire, you are losing precious fluid along with salts that maintain a delicate electrolyte balance in your body. Most off-the-shelf sports drinks can actually do more harm than good because of their high sugar content and unpronounceable list of chemical laden ingredients! We look for a natural, low-sugar sports drink and consume it whenever we are engaging in an activity that results in a lot of perspiration.

Again, there are a wide variety of available products on the market. Do your research and find products you like and use them to take your fitness to the next level.

CHAPTER NINETEEN

Next Level Lifestyle

Deb's Story: When I was working in the construction industry as a "green building" inspector, I had occasion to participate in trade shows where the focus was eco-friendly housing. In 2008, I was at one of these events with my oldest daughter, Erin. While I was working in our booth, Erin walked around looking at what the other exhibitors had to offer. She met a representative from a health and wellness company who got her thinking about chemical free cleaning products. Erin pestered me once we got home until I agreed to purchase a pack of the products. Our deal was contingent on her removing all the existing cleaning products from our home AND doing all the household cleaning with the new products, because, frankly, I didn't believe they would work and didn't want to be bothered.

To my surprise we found that these natural cleaning products (both household cleaners and laundry detergents) worked great – even better than their chemical cousins! As I researched what I had purchased, I was appalled by what I was reading and I started thinking that perhaps getting all the chemicals out of the house might actually help my medical conditions.

Over time I found that I became really sensitive even to the smell of our old household cleaners which were stored in our garage. We threw away all of the old, store-bought products and have not looked back.

Use Nontoxic Household Cleaners and Laundry Detergents: Standard household cleaning and laundry products may contain chemicals such as chlorine, phthalates and volatile organic compounds, or VOCs, to name only a few. Chlorinated materials break down into organochlorine compounds, which are stored in human fat cells and tissues. Phthalates, often used to add fragrance to cleaning solutions, are known to cause reproductive toxicity and disrupt the endocrine system. The Environmental Protection Agency (EPA) warns against VOCs as being suspected of causing cancer! The EPA also found that the levels of some organics are often two to five times greater indoors than outdoors. By avoiding commercial cleaning products that contain these chemicals, you can protect yourself from unnecessary exposure and illness. Additionally, most cleaning compounds employ the use of surfactants, chemicals that help to dissolve and release grease and grime. However, a family of surfactants known as nonylphenols is particularly bad for the environment. These chemicals actually become more toxic as they break down, and they take the longest to disintegrate. This prolonged time in the environment damages water quality and threatens organisms. As if all this weren't enough, every year Poison Control Centers nationwide receive reports of more than two million poisonings. Families with small children can better protect them by replacing dangerous chemicals with nontoxic alternatives.

There are so many wonderful, nontoxic household cleaning and laundry products that perform amazingly well and are safe for people and the environment. WE urge you to take the time and find the ones that work for you.

CHAPTER TWENTY

This is Just the Beginning

You have reached the end of this book, but it is just the beginning of your *Release* journey. Embrace *Release* as a lifestyle – not just the Body section, but especially the Mind and Spirit sections, because THAT is where the recipe for true transformation can be found – not just in your physical body, but in every aspect of your life – personal, professional, financial, spiritual and beyond! You really do have the power to create the life you want to live. You have read our stories. There is nothing remarkable about either of us – we are just two women who got sick of settling for the leftovers of life and decided to make our own path. You can do that too. It is simple – we've shown you that – but it is not necessarily easy! Sometimes you need help and support along the way and that's what we are here for.

We don't want to see you get "most of the way there." We want to see you transform every area of your life that you wish to change!! That's why we offer you continued and on-going guidance with our "My *Release* Plan" online membership. It's an online repository of all things related to the *Release* Plan – extra meal plans, recipes, workouts, articles, product recommendations, blogs, plus with our Premium Membership you receive personal weekly lessons from us to keep you focused on your goal (get an upgrade to the Premium Membership FREE for 30 days at *MyReleasePlan.com*). And once per month you'll have access to a live conference call where we will teach on a particular topic related to Mind, Body or Spirit. It is a phenomenal resource!

Congratulations again for taking this step and creating the body and the life that you truly deserve!!

In addition to My *Release* Plan, we also love to spread this information as far and wide as we can. We would love to speak to your group, company, conference or convention to share this message. Contact our offices at (386) 308-1804 or by email at release@myreleaseplan.com for more information.

Deb Cheslow & Angie Flynn

Deb Cheslow Consulting, is a developmental corporate training company that focuses on helping teams and corporations increase , not only the health and wellness of its employees through our corporate wellness programs, but also thei productivity and efficiency, while facilitating the return on investment of previously spent training program dollars. We provide the tools, systems and ongoing support you need to empower your employees to actually implement the information they already possess.

It is our contention that the people who work within your organization don't require additional training on the particulars of how to do their job, but rather require an actual transformation in their thinking with regard to everything in their lives – including their function within the company. Your company's employees already know everything they need to do in order to do their job productively, efficiently and effectively – but they don't DO it – not with dependable regularity.

Our customized approach goes to the core of this "information-action gap." Our trainers expertly guide each participant on a journey where they discover why they do what they do (and, equally as important, why they don't do what they know they should do) and moreover, empower them with the tools required to bring their desires and their results into complete congruency, both in their personal and professional lives! Your people are your organization's greatest resource and our programs provide the very best information available worldwide on how to draw the most out of each and every one of them, based upon your training objectives.

Contact us today to learn more about our customized corporate training programs or to book Deb Cheslow to speak at your next meeting or convention at (386) 308-2155 or by email at info@ debcheslow.com.

Appendix

Deb Cheslow & Angie Flynn

Appendix A

Resources

MyReleasePlan.com – Extensive resources to keep you on your *Release* path. Weekly emails designed to keep you moving forward in aligning your self-image with the person you truly desire to be, meal plans and recipes, exercise tips, blogs, recommended resources – your one stop solution!

Body for Life, Bill Phillips and Michael d'Orso, William Morrow; 1st edition (June 10, 1999) – Available at major booksellers or online: Excellent commentary on philosophy behind interval training, with sample workouts for both High-Intensity Interval Training and strength training.

Eating for Life, Bill Phillips. High Point Media, Golden, CO. 2003. Available at major booksellers or online: Fantastic menu planning resource. Over 150 recipes for Breakfast, Lunch, Dinner, snacks and desserts that are delicious and fit the guidelines of the *Release* program.

Pinterest.com – We found this image driven social media site an incredible resource for finding pictures to build vision boards or computer screensavers. Searchable by category, you can find anything from a headless body with perfect 6-pack abs to healthy recipes to motivational quotations.

Deb Cheslow & Angie Flynn

Appendix B

14-Day Meal Plan & Recipes

*"You were born to win, but to be a winner, you must plan
to win, prepare to win, and expect to win."*
–Zig Ziglar

Deb Cheslow & Angie Flynn

14-Day Sample Meal Plan

The following menus are designed to give you ideas for meals. They can be mixed and matched however you see fit. We've included meals that need little or no preparation at all (like an apple and a couple of pieces of string cheese) and recipes that require some more advanced culinary skill (nothing terribly difficult, but certainly more advanced than grabbing an apple and some cheese from the fridge) and are absolutely appropriate for a dinner party. And then there is everything in between. You can also see 90+ Days of Angie's meal plans (including what she ate on free days) at *MyReleasePlan.com*. The meal plans below are only ideas – play with your food, learn to love cooking and eating! This is a lifestyle, not a "diet." ENJOY!!!

There are a few things to keep in mind as you go through this section.

1. Although the *Release* Plan is not about counting every calorie that goes into your mouth, we have included the calorie count for the recipes so you can get an idea of what a typical meal consists of.
2. The nutritional information given is based upon a single serving of that recipe.
3. This 14 day menu is designed to show variety. In reality, we would never work that hard!! Pick 2-3 meals and repeat them throughout the week – remember, cook once, eat twice (or thrice).
4. You may drink water, black coffee or tea with each meal – preferably water. Remember, each cup of coffee requires the consumption of an equal amount of water.

Sunday
Breakfast: Meal Replacement Shake
Snack: Ham, egg and cheese muffin
Lunch: Roast Beef and Horseradish Wrap
Snack: Peanut Butter Cup Shake
Dinner: Basil-Garlic Stuffed Chicken, Brown Rice, Peas
Snack: Protein Shake (soy or whey protein)

Monday
Breakfast: Meal Replacement Shake,
Snack: Protein Oatmeal
Lunch: Tuna Salad Wrap
Snack: Apple with Peanut Butter
Dinner: Baked Pesto Chicken, Orzo, Broccol
Snack: Protein Shake (soy or whey protein)

Tuesday
Breakfast: Meal Replacement Shake
Snack: Ham, Egg and Cheese Potato
Lunch: BBQ Chicken Pita Pizza
Snack: Apple with String Cheese
Dinner: Fish Tacos, Guacamole
Snack: Protein Shake (soy or whey protein)

Wednesday
Breakfast: Meal Replacement Shake
Snack: Eggs and Granola
Lunch: Turkey/Ham Sandwich
Snack: (2) Double Chocolate Muffin (or 1 jumbo muffin)
Dinner: Turkey Stuffed Portobello Mushrooms, Smashed Potatoes,
Green Beans, water
Snack: Protein Shake (soy or whey protein)

Thursday
Breakfast: Meal Replacement Shake
Snack: Greek Yogurt Parfait with Fruit and Granola
Lunch: Greek Pita Pizza
Snack: High Protein Snack Bar
Dinner: Chili-Rubbed Tilapia, Brown Rice, Steamed Asparagus,
water
Snack: Protein Shake (soy or whey protein)

Friday
Breakfast: Meal Replacement Shake
Snack: Hard-Boiled Eggs and Whole Wheat Toast
Lunch: Turkey Burger
Snack: Chai-Protein Latte

Dinner: Honey-Soy Salmon, Sweet Potato, Sauteed Spinach
Snack: Protein Shake (soy or whey protein)

Saturday
FREE DAY

Sunday
Breakfast: Meal Replacement Shake
Snack: Spinach Frittata with Toast
Lunch: Tuna Salad with Wheat Thins
Snack: (2) Hard-Boiled Eggs and an Orange
Dinner: Grilled Chicken Bruschetta, Whole Wheat Orzo,
Sauteed Zucchini
Snack: Protein Shake (soy or whey protein)

Monday
Breakfast: Meal Replacement Shake
Snack: Oat Bran Muffin
Lunch: Salmon Salad Sandwich
Snack: Cottage Cheese and Tomatoes
Dinner: Tex-Mex Casserole
Snack: Protein Shake (soy or whey protein)

Tuesday
Breakfast: Meal Replacement Shake
Snack: Denver Omelette
Lunch: Pizza Burger
Snack: Brownie Surprise
Dinner: Stuffed Peppers
Snack: Protein Shake (soy or whey protein)

Wednesday
Breakfast: Meal Replacement Shake
Snack: Mixed Berry Smoothie
Lunch: Creamy Tarragon Chicken Salad
Snack: English Muffin Pizza
Dinner: Sesame-Herb Crusted Mahi-Mahi, Brown Rice, Spinach
Snack: Protein Shake (soy or whey protein)

Thursday
Breakfast: Meal Replacement Shake
Snack: Vanilla-Peanut Butter Smoothie
Lunch: BBQ Chicken Sandwich
Snack: Chocolate Pudding
Dinner: Chicken Enchiladas
Snack: Protein Shake (soy or whey protein)

Friday
Breakfast: Meal Replacement Shake
Snack: Bagel with Smoked Salmon and Cream Cheese
Lunch: Cashew-Chicken Salad, Light Salad Dressing
Snack: Cheese Quesadilla
Dinner: Flank Steak Pinwheels, Mashed Potatoes, Steamed Asparagus
Snack: Protein Shake (soy or whey protein)

Saturday
FREE DAY

Recipes

All of the recipes are intended to be quick and easy to prepare with ingredients you can find in any decent supermarket. We are extremely busy, on-the-go people – especially Deb, who is with clients during the day – and our meal plans have to consist of food we can pack and take with us. Angie loves to cook, but that said, leaves the meals that require a lot of prep time for the weekends. Our average weekday dinner can be prepped in less than 15 minutes and cooked in 20-30 minutes. ENJOY!!

Breakfasts

Ham, Egg and Cheese Muffin
*Who needs McDonald's when you can whip up this breakfast classic in a flash – only **this** version is good for you!!*

1 whole wheat English muffin
1 large egg
½ Tbsp water
1 slice 2% cheddar cheese
2 slices Nitrite-Free Ham (like Hormel Natural Choice)

Toast English muffin to desired darkness. Preheat a small skillet lightly sprayed with olive oil spray. While muffin is toasting, whisk egg and water together until frothy. Pour into preheated skillet and cook eggs until set. Transfer eggs to one half of toasted English muffin and top with cheese slice. Warm ham slices in skillet and place on top of cheese. Add muffin top and enjoy!

Recipe makes 1 serving
290 Calories; 11 g Total Fat; 27 g Carbohydrate; 3 g Fiber; 21 g Protein

Protein Packed Oatmeal
This oatmeal is wonderfully satisfying on a cool morning and has real staying power with the added protein. You can also mix it up by adding chocolate or vanilla favored protein powder – YUMMY!!

½ cup water
Dash of salt
¼ cup old-fashioned oats
10 raisins
3 Tbsp plain protein powder (soy or whey)
¼ tsp cinnamon
½ cup skim milk

Bring water and salt to a boil in a small pan, stir in oats and reduce heat to low. Cover. Cook for 5 minutes and remove from heat. Stir in raisins, protein powder and cinnamon. Transfer to a small bowl and add milk. Stir and serve.

Recipe makes 1 serving
241 Calories; 3 g Total Fat; 34 g Carbohydrate; 2 g Fiber; 21 g Protein

Ham and Egg Baked Potato
Great on-the-go breakfast – hearty and delicious – and a fantastic way to use up leftover baked potatoes.

1 russet potato (fist sized)
1 egg
½ slice Nitrite-free Ham
1 Tbsp Shredded Cheddar cheese

Bake potato in either the microwave oven (~5 minutes) or conventional oven (~45 minutes at 450°F). Carefully slice off the top and scoop out the inside to make a bowl – leave sides ~1/4 inch thick. Place ham in bottom of potato "bowl", then crack egg inside and top with cheese. Bake at 350°F for 25 minutes or until egg is set.

Recipe makes 1 serving
212 calories; 9 g Total Fat; 19 g Carbohydrate; 1 g Fiber; 12 g Protein

Eggs and Cereal
Cheesy scrambled eggs with multi-grain cereal (we like french vanilla granola)

2 large eggs
1 Tbsp water
1-1/2 Tbsp 2% shredded cheddar cheese
½ cup granola (or 1 serving of other low sugar, multigrain cereal)
½ cup skim milk

Lightly spray a nonstick skillet with olive oil spray and preheat to medium. Whisk eggs and water in a bowl until smooth and frothy. Pour eggs into skillet. As they begin to set, use a spatula to lift cooked portions, allowing uncooked egg to flow underneath. Cook until eggs are set, 3-4 minutes. When eggs are set, sprinkle cheese over top and slide onto a plate. Pour cereal into a bowl and top with skim milk. Serve immediately.

Recipe makes 1 serving
399 calories (with granola as the cereal); 13 g Total Fat; 19 g Carbohydrate; 1 g Fiber; 21 g Protein

Greek Yogurt Parfait with Fruit and Granola
Greek yogurt has substantially more protein than regular yogurt and gives this tasty breakfast real staying power!

½ cup nonfat vanilla greek yogurt
½ cup fruit (you can mix and match fruits, but no more than ½ cup total – we like blueberries and grapes)
2 Tbsp granola

You can get fancy and layer the ingredients in one of those cool parfait glasses or just serve in a cereal bowl like we do.

Recipe makes 1 parfait
191 Calories; 1 g Total Fat; 22 g Carbohydrate; 1 g Fiber; 12 g Protein

Hard-Boiled Eggs and Toast
Easy grab and go breakfast that sticks with you. Hint: Make several days worth of hard-boiled eggs at once, so breakfast on those out of control busy days is a no-brainer.

2 large eggs, hard-boiled (see Helpful Hint)
1 slice Ezekiel bread

1 tsp. Concord grape jelly
Salt and pepper to taste

Remove shells from eggs. Toast bread and spread 1 tsp of jelly on slice. You can salt and pepper eggs to your preferred taste.

Recipe makes 1 serving
237 Calories; 8 g Total Fat; 20 g Carbohydrate; 3 g Fiber; 16 g Protein

---

Helpful Hint: Perfect Hard-Boiled Eggs

Place eggs in a pot and cover with water (about 1" above eggs). Cover pot and bring water to a slow boil, then reduce heat to low and simmer for 15 minutes. Drain water and refill pan with cold water. Add ice to water to chill eggs even faster.

Spinach Frittata with Toast
This is a great option for brunch. Just add a slice of toast per person and you have a wonderfully filling and delicious meal!

1 tsp. extra-virgin olive oil
4 large eggs
4 egg whites
2 Tbsp. water
¼ tsp. salt
¼ tsp. freshly ground black pepper
10 oz. frozen, chopped spinach, thawed and drained well (see Helpful Hint below)
¼ cup reduced fat crumbled feta cheese
1 cup grape tomatoes, halved
3 oz part-skim mozzarella cheese, shredded
3 scallions, chopped

Preheat oven to 400°F.

In a mixing bowl, whisk together eggs, egg whites, water, salt and pepper. Set aside.

Heat oil to medium in an oven proof, non-stick skillet. Sauté scallions until translucent, about 4-5 minutes. Add spinach and mix in with onions. Spread out spinach mixture evenly on bottom of skillet. Pour egg mixture over spinach. Use a spatula to lift up the spinach mixture along the sides of the pan to let egg mixture flow underneath.

Arrange grape tomato halves over top of egg mixture and sprinkle with feta cheese. When the mixture is about halfway set, put the whole pan in the oven. Bake for 10 minutes, frittata will still be loose in the center. Sprinkle with mozzarella cheese and return to oven for 5 minutes longer until cheese is melted and frittata is puffy and golden. Remove from oven with oven mitts and let cool for several minutes. CAUTION: The skillet handle will be HOT!!!

Cut into quarters and serve with a slice of whole wheat toast.

Recipe makes 4 servings
275 Calories; 11.5 g Total Fat; 20 g Carbohydrate; 4 g Fiber; 23 g Protein

Helpful Hint: Draining Spinach

Frozen spinach is one of the most versatile ingredients in the supermarket, an incredible value and is amazingly good for you! Low in calories and high in vitamins, spinach is one of the most nutrient-dense foods in existence. One cup of the leafy green vegetable contains far more than your daily requirements of vitamin K and vitamin A, almost all the manganese and folate your body needs and nearly 40 percent of your magnesium requirement. It is a good, very good or excellent source of more than 20 different measurable nutrients, including dietary fiber, calcium and protein. And yet, 1 cup has only 40 calories! The only problem is that it holds a lot of water, which can be a problem in some recipes. This can easily be dealt with though. Thaw spinach in the box or bag and then dump into a colander. Now take the spinach in your hand or place in a clean kitchen towel and squeeze all the excess water out of it. The resulting product will be dry wilted spinach leaves ready to be added to your favorite recipe!

Deb Cheslow & Angie Flynn

Deb's Oat Bran Muffins

A moist and tasty grab and go breakfast or snack. Especially good warm with a touch of maple syrup!!

1 cup oat bran
1 cup nonfat powdered milk
¼ + 1/8 tsp baking soda
1 Tbsp. ground cinnamon
1 Tbsp. vanilla extract
6 packets Truvia sweetener
1-1/2 cups Egg Beaters
2 scoops vanilla protein powder (soy or whey)
1-1/2 cup unsweetened applesauce

Preheat oven to 350°F.

Line muffin pan with jumbo foil muffin cup liners and lightly spray with nonstick cooking spray.

Mix all ingredients together in a large bowl until well combined. Spoon into prepared muffin liners (almost all the way to the top). Bake in preheated oven for 20-25 minutes or until a toothpick inserted in the center of a muffin comes out clean.

Recipe makes ~8 servings (1 jumbo muffin per serving)
317 Calories; 4 g Total Fat; 59 g Carbohydrate; 10 g Fiber; 24 g Protein

Denver Omelet

A one-pan meal – eggs, potatoes, ham, veggies – all in one. Delicious, hearty comfort food!

2 large eggs
1 Tbsp water
¼ cup cubed, frozen hash brown potatoes
¼ cup chopped bell pepper
1 Tbsp chopped red onion
2 oz Nitrite-free deli ham, chopped
2 Tbsp, 2% cheddar cheese, shredded

Spray a small nonstick skillet with nonstick cooking spray and preheat to medium.

Crack eggs into a small bowl, add water and beat with a fork or a whisk until fluffy.

Add peppers and onion and sauté 2-3 minutes, add potatoes and continue to sauté until onions are translucent (another 2-3 minutes). Add ham. Add egg mixture to the pan.

Use a spatula to lift and allow eggs to flow underneath. Repeat this until eggs are set. If firmer eggs are desired, you can place the skillet under the broiler for 1-2 minutes. Add cheese and turn out onto a plate, allowing omelet to fold in half.

Recipe makes 1 serving
242 Calories; 12 g Total Fat; 9 g Carbohydrate; 1 g Fiber; 21 g Protein

Mixed Berry Smoothie
Thick rich smoothie tastes like a free-day milkshake!

½ cup frozen blueberries
4 large frozen strawberries
1 cup skim milk
1 scoop vanilla protein powder (soy or whey)

Place all ingredients in a blender and process until smooth. Pour into a cup and add a straw!

Recipe makes 1 serving
308 Calories; 2 g Total Fat; 42 g Carbohydrate; 3 g Fiber; 31 g Protein

Bagel with Cream Cheese and Lox
We love to have bagels and lox with all the fixins for a Free Day breakfast or brunch every now and then. With this version, you can enjoy it any day!

1 Thomas' Light Bagel or 1/2 of a Thomas' Whole Wheat Bagel
1 Tbsp. Light Cream Cheese

Deb Cheslow & Angie Flynn

2 oz. smoked salmon
2 slices tomato
1 slice red onion
1 tsp nonpareil capers

Slice bagel in half and toast. Spread ½ Tbsp of cream cheese on each bagel half. Layer 1 oz smoked salmon, 1 tomato slice and a couple of rings of red onion on top of cream cheese. Sprinkle each half with capers.

Recipe makes 1 serving
308 Calories; 10 g Total Fat; 43 g Carbohydrate; 14 g Fiber; 24 g Protein

Vanilla Peanut Butter Smoothie
So delicious it feels like a "cheat," but it's a GREAT breakfast or snack on the Release Plan!

1 cup skim milk
1 Tbsp. natural peanut butter
1 scoop vanilla meal replacement shake mix
8 ice cubes

Place all ingredients in a blender and process until smooth. Pour into a glass and add straw! Enjoy!!

Recipe makes 1 serving
305 Calories; 10 g Total Fat; 17 g Carbohydrate; 1 g Fiber; 35 g Protein

Lunches

Roast Beef and Horseradish Wrap
A delicious deli classic

1 Tbsp. light mayonnaise
1 tsp. prepared horseradish
4 oz. Nitrite-Free Deli Roast Beef (like Dietz and Watson)
1 romaine lettuce leaf
1 thick slice tomato, cut in half
1 Large La Tortilla Factory Whole Wheat Tortilla

Mix mayo and horseradish in a small bowl and spread on half of tortilla. Place roast beef over tortilla. Top with lettuce and tomato. Tuck in sides and roll. Cut in half and enjoy.

Recipe makes 1 serving
283 Calories; 11 g Total Fat; 22 g Carbohydrate; 13 g Fiber; 32 g Protein

Tuna Salad Wrap
Great on-the-go lunch.

1 3-oz can solid white albacore tuna packed in water, drained
1 Tbsp. light mayonnaise
1 Tbsp. chopped celery
1 Tbsp. chopped onion
2 tsp. sweet pickle relish
1 Large La Tortilla Factory Whole Wheat tortilla
1 Romaine lettuce leaf
1 thick slice of tomato cut in half

Mix first 5 ingredients in a bowl until well combined. Spread on half of tortilla.

Top with lettuce and tomato. Roll into wrap.

Recipe makes 1 wrap sandwich
198 Calories; 8 g Total Fat; 22 g Carbohydrate; 12 g Fiber; 18 g Protein

BBQ Chicken Pita Pizza

Delicious crispy pita crust topped with BBQ sauce, chicken breast, red onion and mozzarella cheese. Yummy!!!

1-1/2 whole wheat pita
1-1/2 Tbsp of your favorite barbeque sauce (less sugar is best)
6 oz cooked chicken breast
1-1/2 slice red onion, diced
1/3 cup 2% fat shredded mozzarella cheese
¼ tsp Italian seasoning

Preheat oven to 425°F. Spread barbeque sauce evenly on top of pitas. Top with chicken, onion and cheese. Sprinkle with Italian seasoning. Place pitas on baking sheet and bake for 10-12 minutes. Slice whole pita into 4 wedges and the half pita into 2 wedges. Serving size is 3 wedges.

Recipe makes 2 servings
292 Calories; 5 g Total Fat; 33 g Carbohydrate; 3 g Fiber; 32 g Protein

Turkey Sandwich

A tad on the obvious side, but always a great go-to lunch. Find nitrite-free deli meats whenever you are able (Hormel Natural Choice Deli Cuts and Dietz & Watson are two great brands).

2 slices Ezekiel Sprouted Wheat Bread
2 oz nitrite-free deli turkey
1 slice 2% cheddar cheese
2 tsp honey mustard
1 slice tomato
1 romaine lettuce leaf

Spread mustard on one slice of bread. Layer turkey, cheese, tomato and lettuce on top of mustard. Top with remaining slice of bread.

Recipe makes 1 serving
282 Calories; 4 g Total Fat; 33 g Carbohydrate; 6 g Fiber; 22 g Protein

Greek Chicken Pita Pizza
We love our pita pizzas!! This version uses hummus as a base and feta cheese in place of mozzarella! It's one of our favorite lunches!!

1-1/2 whole wheat pitas
3 Tbsp hummus (any variety)
6 oz chicken breast, diced
1-1/2 slice red onion
¼ cup roasted red pepper, sliced into strips
½ cup crumbled feta cheese
¼ tsp Italian seasoning

Preheat oven to 425°F. Spread pitas evenly with hummus. Top with chicken, onion and peppers. Sprinkle evenly with crumbled feta cheese and Italian seasoning. Place pitas on baking sheet and bake for 10-12 minutes. Slice whole pita into 4 wedges and the half pita into 2 wedges. Serving size is 3 wedges.

Recipe makes 2 servings
305 Calories; 8 g Total Fat; 32 g Carbohydrate; 5 g Fiber; 30 g Protein

Turkey Burger
We adapted this recipe from the book Eating for Life which is a fantastic resource for recipes that fit the Release program (see RESOURCES section). This burger is very flavorful and the perfect lunch!!

1 lb. lean ground turkey breast
½ onion, finely diced
2 tsp horseradish
1 tsp low-sodium soy sauce
2 cloves minced garlic
3 large, organic eggs
4 whole wheat hamburger buns
4 Romaine lettuce leaves
4 thick slices of tomato
Ketchup and/or mustard as you like it

Preheat broiler to High (or preheat grill). In a large bowl, combine turkey, onion, horseradish, soy sauce, garlic and eggs. Form into 4 equal sized patties. Place on a foil lined baking pan and broil for 5 minutes, turn over and broil for an additional 5 minutes or until burger is no longer pink inside.

Place burger on whole-wheat bun with lettuce, tomato and condiments.

Recipe makes 4 burgers
227 Calories; 3 g Total Fat; 30 g Carbohydrate; 5 g Fiber; 23 g Protein

---

Helpful Hint: Lean Ground Turkey Breast vs. Regular Ground Turkey vs. Frozen Ground Turkey

When perusing your local supermarket's meat section, you will likely find several forms of ground turkey – lean ground turkey breast, regular ground turkey and frozen ground turkey. Lean ground turkey breast is, as its name implies, the breast meat of the turkey ground up and contains only ~1% fat. Regular ground turkey is made from white and dark meat with some skin, and is about 10% fat (similar to ground round). Frozen ground turkey is usually all dark meat with skin, and is 15% fat, similar to ground sirloin. It may be tempting from a budgetary stance to purchase the less expensive frozen ground turkey or the regular ground turkey from the meat case, but do yourself a favor and stick with the ground turkey breast. All the *Release* Plan recipes that include turkey, specify lean ground turkey breast.

Tuna Salad and Wheat Thins
Simple, filling and tasty – a great on the go lunch

1 3-oz can solid white albacore tuna packed in water, drained
1 Tbsp. light mayonnaise
1 Tbsp. chopped celery
1 Tbsp. chopped onion

2 tsp. sweet pickle relish
1 serving of Wheat Thin crackers

Mix first 5 ingredients in a small bowl. Let chill for at least one hour. Serve on wheat thins.

Recipe makes 1 serving
338 Calories; 14 g Total Fat; 25 g Carbohydrate; 1 g Fiber; 25 g Protein

Salmon Salad Sandwich
This recipe is even better when you prepare it with leftover Honey-Soy Salmon filets (see Dinner section), but the canned salmon is very good as well and very convenient.

1 14.75 oz. can boneless, skinless wild Alaskan salmon, drained
¼ cup minced red onion
2 Tbsp. lemon juice
1 Tbsp. extra-virgin olive oil
¼ tsp. freshly ground black pepper
4 Tbsp. lowfat cream cheese
8 slices pumpernickel bread, toasted
8 slices tomato
4 leaves romaine lettuce

Combine salmon, onion, lemon juice, olive oil and pepper in a medium sized bowl. Spread 1 Tbsp of the cream cheese on each of 4 slices of the bread. Spread ½ cup of salmon salad over the cream cheese. Top each sandwich half with 2 slices of tomato, a lettuce leaf and another slice of bread.

Recipe makes 4 servings
374 Calories; 13 g Total Fat; 35 g Carbohydrate; 3 g Fiber; 25 g Protein

Pizza Burger
Inspired by a free day favorite, this burger is savory, satisfying and absolute plan PERFECT!

1 lb. lean ground turkey breast
1-1/2 cup organic marinara sauce, divided

¼ cup grated parmesan cheese
1 Tbsp. Italian seasoning
2 tsp. Dijon mustard
4 slices part-skim mozzarella cheese
1/3 cup fresh basil, chopped
4 lite whole wheat hamburger buns, toasted if desired

Preheat grill or broiler to high.

In a large mixing bowl add turkey breast, ½ cup of marinara sauce, parmesan cheese, Italian seasoning, and Dijon mustard. Mix until well combined.

Line a baking sheet with aluminum foil and spray lightly with nonstick cooking spray. Divide turkey mixture into 4 equal portions and shape each into a patty and place on baking sheet.

Broil or grill patties until cooked through, approximately 6 minutes per side. Top burgers with remaining marinara sauce and one slice of cheese each and continue cooking until cheese is melted.

Transfer each burger to one half of a toasted bun. Top with remaining half.

Recipe makes 4 servings
410 Calories; 11 g Total Fat; 28 g Carbohydrate, 4 g Fiber; 46 g Protein

Creamy Tarragon Chicken Salad
Great "prepare once, eat all week" recipe.

2 lb. boneless, skinless chicken breasts
1 cup reduced sodium chicken broth
1/3 cup walnuts, rough chopped
2/3 cup light sour cream
½ cup light mayonnaise
¼ cup fresh tarragon, chopped (1 Tbsp dry tarragon can be substituted)
¼ tsp. salt
½ tsp. freshly ground black pepper

1-1/2 cups celery, diced
1-1/2 cups seedless red grapes, halved

Preheat oven to 450°F.

Arrange chicken in single layer in a glass baking dish. Pour broth around chicken. Bake chicken until no longer pink in the center (internal temperature of 170°F), 30-35 minutes. Allow chicken to cool until you can handle it, then cut into cubes. Discard broth.

Meanwhile spread walnuts on a clean baking sheet and toast in oven until golden and fragrant, about 6 minutes. Let cool.

In a large bowl, mix together sour cream, mayonnaise, tarragon, salt and pepper. Add celery, grapes, chicken and walnuts. Stir until well combined and evenly coated. Refrigerate until chilled (at least 1 hour).

Recipe makes 8 (1 cup) servings
231 Calories; 11 g Total Fat; 9 g Carbohydrate; 1 g Fiber; 26 g Protein

BBQ Chicken Sandwich
A great recipe to use up leftover chicken breast! So easy to make and so tasty!!

½ cup cooked chicken breast, shredded
¼ cup carrots, shredded
2 Tbsp barbeque sauce
2 tsp. light ranch dressing
1 lite whole wheat hamburger bun

Toss chicken, carrots and barbeque sauce in a small bowl to combine and microwave on HIGH for 1 minute until hot. Spread ranch dressing on half of hamburger bun. Top with chicken mixture and other half of bun. Enjoy!

Recipe makes 1 serving
286 Calories; 5 g Total Fat; 37 g Carbohydrate; 5 g Fiber; 26 g Protein

Deb Cheslow & Angie Flynn

Cashew-Chicken Salad

Great option for lunch or dinner. Grilled chicken, hard-boiled egg, and cashews make this a very hearty salad!

2 cups chopped Romaine lettuce
½ medium cucumber, sliced
¼ tomato, sliced (or chopped, or wedged – whatever)
1 slice red onion, separated into rings
1 hard-boiled egg, cut into quarters
2 oz. chicken breast, diced or shredded
1 Tbsp. cashews, roughly chopped
2 Tbsp. 2% cheddar cheese, shredded
2 Tbsp. of your favorite light salad dressing

Layer ingredients in order on a dinner plate. Drizzle with dressing. Add fork.

Recipe makes 1 serving
296 Calories; 14 g Total Fat; 29 g Carbohydrate; 3 g Fiber; 21.5 g Protein

Snacks

Peanut Butter Cup Shake
Delicious, cool, filling treat – ready in a jiffy!

1 cup skim milk
2 scoops chocolate meal replacement mix
1 tbsp natural peanut butter
6-8 ice cubes

Place all ingredients in a blender and blend on high until smooth. Pour in a cup, add a straw and enjoy!

Recipe makes 1 serving
280 Calories; 10 g Total Fat; 28 g Carbohydrate; 4 g Fiber; 20 g Protein

Apple and Peanut Butter
It doesn't get any more basic or easy – slices of apple spread with natural peanut butter – simple, filling and delicious! This is one of our favorite snacks for taking on the road with us – especially when we are flying. Super simple and portable!!

1 fist-sized apple
2 Tbsp natural peanut butter (creamy or chunky)

Slice apple into wedges, spread with or dip into peanut butter and eat.

Recipe makes 1 serving
285 Calories; 16 g Total Fat; 22 g Carbohydrate; 4 g Fiber; 8 g Protein

Apple and String Cheese
Another quick and easy go-to snack when we're on the road.

1 fist-sized apple
2 2% reduced fat string cheese

Eat and enjoy!!

Recipe makes 1 serving

Deb Cheslow & Angie Flynn

215 Calories; 12 g Total Fat; 18 g Carbohydrate; 2 g Fiber; 14 g Protein

Triple Chocolate Muffin

If you love those VitaTop muffins in the freezer section of the health food store, you will go crazy over these! Just as good, easy and freeze really well, so make a double batch and freeze for a grab and go snack any time!

1-3/4 cups Quaker old-fashioned oatmeal
3 large egg whites
2/3 cup unsweetened cocoa powder
1/2 cup unsweetened applesauce
1 tsp vanilla extract
1/2 cup plain nonfat Greek yogurt
1/2 tsp cream of tartar
1-1/2 tsp baking powder
1-1/2 tsp baking soda
1/4 tsp salt
1 cup hot water
1 cup granular splenda
1/4 cup semi-sweet mini chocolate chips
3 scoops chocolate protein powder (whey or soy)

Preheat oven to 350 degrees.

Line (12-cup) muffin pans with foil cupcake liners, or spray muffin tin with non-stick cooking spray. Set aside.

In a food processor with blade attachment in place, process the oatmeal until the texture of coarse flour. Add all of the remaining ingredients together, except for the chocolate chips, to the food processor bowl. Blend until oats are ground and mixture is smooth. Place mixture in a bowl and gently stir in 1/2 of the chocolate chips (set the rest aside). Scoop mixture into prepared muffin pans. Sprinkle remaining chocolate chips on top of batter in each muffin cup.

Place muffins tins in the oven for 15 minutes , or until a toothpick inserted in the center of a muffin comes out clean.

Cool muffins before removing from pan. ENJOY!!!

Recipe makes 6 servings (2 regular muffins or 1 jumbo muffin = 1 serving)
208 Calories; 6 g Total Fat; 30 g Carbohydrate; 6 g Fiber; 18 g Protein

Protein Snack Bar
Choose a snack bar that has approximately equal amounts of carbohydrate and protein (at least 10 grams per bar), under 4 grams of total fat, and under 200 calories.

Chai-Protein Latte
Like an iced chai latte from a coffee/tea house – only it's great for you!!

½ cup chai tea concentrate
½ cup skim milk (you can also use soy milk or almond milk)
1 scoop vanilla protein powder (soy or whey)
1 cup crushed ice

Combine first 3 ingredients in a blender or shaker cup and mix well. Add crushed ice to a tall glass and pour chai mixture over ice.

Recipe makes 1 serving
210 Calories; 2 g Total Fat; 32 g Carbohydrate; <1 g Fiber; 28 g Protein

Hard-Boiled Eggs and Orange
Perfect for days when you just have to grab something and head out the door. Prepare a dozen eggs at once and you have snacks all week!

2 eggs, hard-boiled
1 medium orange

Peel eggs, add a little salt and pepper if desired. Cut orange into eighths, or just peel and eat.

Recipe makes 1 serving

202 Calories; 10 g Total Fat; 15 g Carbohydrate; 3 g Fiber; 15 g Protein

Cottage Cheese and Tomato
Angie grew up in southwestern Virginia and this was a favorite snack that she would often have with her Grandmother, Ruby Mathena. It was usually accompanied by one of her famous buttermilk biscuits, but we'll save THAT for a Free Day!

½ cup fat-free cottage cheese
1 medium tomato, cut into wedges
1/8 tsp salt
1/8 tsp freshly ground black pepper

Place tomato wedges on a small plate, top with cottage cheese, sprinkle with salt and pepper.

Recipe makes 1 serving
215 Calories; 4 g Total Fat; 24 g Carbohydrate; 2 g Fiber; 17 g Protein

English Muffin Pizza
This is a fantastic snack! The recipe calls for baking the pizza in the oven, but if you are at work and don't have access to an oven you could certainly use a microwave. You can also play with toppings too – we like to add nitrite-free ham and pineapple tidbits!

1 whole wheat English muffin, separated into 2 halves
2 Tbsp. pizza sauce (or spaghetti sauce will work fine too)
2 Tbsp. fat-free cottage cheese
2 Tbsp. part-skim mozzarella cheese, shredded
Preheat oven to 350°F.

Lightly toast English muffin. Spread 1 Tbsp sauce on each half of muffin. Top with 1 Tbsp. cottage cheese and 1 Tbsp. mozzarella cheese on each half. Bake pizzas on a baking sheet for approximately 10 minutes. Serve hot.

Recipe makes 1 serving
200 Calories; 5 g Total Fat; 28 g Carbohydrate; 3 g Fiber; 13 g

Protein

SURPRISE Brownies
Rich chocolatey brownies that have a special, unexpected ingredient!

5 large eggs
½ cup + 6 tsp granulated Splenda, divided
4 Tbsp unsweetened cocoa powder
2 scoops chocolate protein powder (soy or whey)
3 Tbsp. strong coffee (or dissolve 1-1/2 Tbsp instant coffee in 1-1/2 Tbsp. hot water)
1 tsp. baking powder
2 Tbsp. extra-virgin olive oil
1-1/2 tsp. vanilla extract
1 15 oz can black beans (drained and rinsed well)
½ cup light sour cream

Preheat oven to 350°F.

Prepare an 8" x 8" baking pan by spraying it with nonstick cooking spray. Place eggs, ½ cup splenda, cocoa powder, protein powder, coffee, baking powder, olive oil, vanilla extract and black beans in a food processor (with blade attachment in place) or blender. Make sure you add the beans last and blend very well, until very smooth and velvety.

Bake for 30 minutes or until a toothpick inserted in the center of the pan comes out clean. Allow to cool before slicing. Cut brownies into (8) 4" x 2" bars.

Mix sour cream and remaining 6 tsp. of Splenda together. Serve one brownie and top with ~ 1 Tbsp. sour cream mixture.

Recipe makes 8 servings.
183 Calories; 8.5 g Total Fat; 14 g Carbohydrate; 1 g Fiber; 14 g Protein

Angie's Chocolate Pudding
"This is AMAZING!" That's what Angie's 9 year old son, Josh, had to say about this rich, creamy treat that's packed with protein!

2 cups fat-free cottage cheese
2 cups skim milk
2 scoops chocolate protein powder (soy or whey)
1 (six-serving) package instant, sugar-free, fat-free pudding mix
Fat-free whipped topping

Place first four ingredients in a blender and process until smooth. Pour into a large bowl and refrigerate until set (30 minutes). Spoon a serving into a bowl and top with 2 Tbsp. whipped topping.

Recipe makes 4 (1 cup) servings
236 Calories; 1 g Total Fat; 24 g Carbohydrate; 0.5 g Fiber; 30.5 g Protein

Cheese Quesadilla
Melted cheese and salsa in a lightly browned tortilla with sour cream! YUM!!

1 large La Tortilla Factory whole wheat tortilla
1/3 cup Mexican cheese blend, shredded
1 Tbsp. light sour cream
2 Tbsp. salsa (as hot as you like it)

Spray a large skillet with nonstick cooking spray and heat to medium. Place tortilla in the pan. Add cheese evenly, covering most of the tortilla. Watch for cheese to melt. Add salsa and spread over cheese. Close quesadilla by folding tortilla in half. Cook until browned and crispy. Flip over and cook other side until browned and crispy.

Cut in 3 wedges and serve with sour cream.

Recipe makes 1 serving
216 Calories; 11 g Total Fat; 21 g Carbohydrate; 12 g Fiber; 18 g Protein

Release

Dinners

Basil and Garlic Stuffed Chicken
Delicate chicken breast rolled around cheese, herbs and roasted peppers.

¼ cup grated Parmesan Cheese
2 tbsp. chopped fresh basil
1 tbsp + 1 tsp extra-virgin olive oil, divided
2 cloves garlic, minced
1/3 cup roasted red pepper, roughly chopped
4 boneless, skinless chicken breasts cutlets
2 tbsp fresh lemon juice

Preheat oven to 350°F.

Combine parmesan cheese, basil, 1 tbsp olive oil, garlic and peppers in a small bowl. Set aside.

Place each chicken cutlet between two pieces of plastic wrap. Using the flat side of a meat mallet, gently pound until each breast is about 1/8" in thickness. Remove and discard plastic wrap.

Spread ¼ of cheese mixture on each chicken breast. Fold in sides of chicken breast and roll up like a burrito. Fasten with wooden toothpicks. Place on a baking sheet.

In a small bowl combine lemon juice and olive oil and brush over chicken. Bake at 350F for 25 minutes or until chicken is no longer pick (internal temperature reaches 170F), brushing occasionally with sauce.

Recipe makes 4 servings
273 Calories; 10 g Total Fat; 2 g Carbohydrate; 1 g Fiber; 41 g Protein

Baked Pesto Chicken with Orzo
So easy and so good!! Deliciously delicate chicken in a basil, garlic pesto served over whole grain orzo pasta.

4 boneless skinless chicken breasts
½ cup basil pesto (any jarred pesto will do)
½ cup shredded low-fat mozzarella cheese
1/3 cup whole grain orzo (dry), prepared according to package directions
1 16 oz. bag frozen broccoli florets, steamed

Preheat oven to 375°F/190°C

Cut chicken breasts into ~4 oz. strips (cut large breasts into 3 strips and smaller breasts into 2). Spray a 9" x 13" baking pan with nonstick cooking spray. Spread ¼ cup of pesto on bottom of baking pan. Lay chicken strips over pesto, then spread remaining ¼ cup of pesto over the chicken strips.

Cover the baking pan with aluminum foil and bake chicken in preheated oven for 25 (chicken should just be cooked through – don't overcook). Remove foil and sprinkle with mozzarella cheese and return to oven (uncovered) and bake for 5 minutes longer.

Serve hot over cooked orzo. Spoon the leftover juice in the pan over the chicken and orzo. Add a vegetable and you have a meal!

Recipe makes 6 servings
380 Calories; 16 g Total Fat; 28 g Carbohydrate; 4 g Fiber; 34 g Protein

Fish Tacos with Guacamole
Healthier than their deep-fried cousins, these fish tacos incorporate grilled, marinated tilapia filets and a wonderfully creamy, chunky guacamole sauce. A family favorite!

6 limes, divided
6 garlic cloves, minced, divided
2 tsp. ground cumin, divided
1-1/2 lbs. tilapia filets
2 medium avocados, pitted and diced
¼ cup diced red onion
½ jalapeno pepper, diced

¼ cup fresh cilantro, chopped
4 LaTortilla Factory Low-Carb Whole Wheat Tortillas (burrito size)
1/3 cup 2% shredded cheddar cheese
Salsa
Low-Fat Sour Cream

Preheat grill to medium (or preheat broiler).

Combine juice of 3 limes, 3 garlic cloves and 1 tsp cumin in a 1 gallon freezer bag and mix together. Add tilapia to bag, seal bag and let marinate in refrigerator for 15-20 minutes (don't go much longer than this or fish will begin to "cook" in the lime juice and it will be mushy).

While fish is marinating, mix juice from remaining 2 limes, remaining 3 garlic cloves, remaining 1 tsp of cumin, diced avocado, onion, jalapeno and cilantro in a mixing bowl. Grill fish until opaque throughout – approximately 5 minutes per side (or broil on high for 10 minutes).

Heat tortillas on grill (~ 30 seconds per side) or in hot oven.

Place a palm sized portion of fish and ~1/4 cup of guacamole in tortilla. Garnish with 1 tbsp cheese, salsa and sour cream.

Recipe makes 4 servings.
434 Calories; 16 g Total Fat; 39 g Carbohydrate; 23 g Fiber; 47 g Protein

---

Helpful Hint: The Easy Way to Dice an Avocado

Step 1- Slice the avocado in half. Twist the two halves a quarter of a turn and lift. The pit will stay with one half.

Step 2- Stick the pit with a knife and pluck it out.

Step 3- Gently take the knife and slice the avocado flesh vertically and horizontally, making a crosshatch pattern (use caution not to pierce the peel, lest you cut your hand).

Step 4- Take a spoon and slide the edge between the flesh and the avocado skin.

Step 5- Scoop out the flesh following the contour of the skin. You will have perfect chunks of avocado with no mess!

Turkey Stuffed Portobello Mushrooms
These stuffed mushrooms are absolutely delicious and satisfying. They hit all those wonderful comfort food pleasure centers. You'll want to double the recipe so you can have leftovers!!

1 tbsp extra-virgin olive oil
1 sweet yellow onion, thinly sliced
2 tsp apple cider vinegar
¾ tsp ground sage
½ tsp fresh rosemary, chopped
½ tsp salt
½ tsp freshly ground black pepper
1/8 tsp ground nutmeg
1 pound lean ground turkey breast
4 large Portobello mushroom caps, gills removed
1 tbsp Worcestershire sauce
½ cup shredded fontina cheese

Position oven rack on lowest position and preheat oven to 400°F/205°C.

Heat oil in a large pan to medium, add onions. Stir occasionally and reduce the heat as necessary to prevent scorching. Cook onions for approximately 20 minutes until they are golden and soft. Stir in vinegar.

In a large bowl knead together turkey, sage, rosemary, salt, pepper, and nutmeg until well combined. Form into 4 equal sized balls.

Remove gills from mushroom caps (see helpful hint) and brush each mushroom on both sides with Worcestershire sauce. Place one turkey in each mushroom cap, patting down to fill the entire cap. Place on a baking sheet.

Bake the stuffed mushrooms for about 20 minutes, until the mushrooms begin to soften. Remove from oven and top each mushroom with ¼ of the onion mixture and ¼ of the shredded cheese. Return baking sheet to oven and continue baking until the cheese is melted and browned and the turkey is complete cooked through (about 10 minutes).

Recipe makes 4 servings
278 Calories; 11.5 g Total Fat; 5.5 g Carbohydrate; 1 g Fiber; 36 g Protein

---

Helpful Hint: Removing the Gills from a Portobello

The gills in a Portobello mushroom are edible, but they are easily removed using a small spoon. Just pull off the remainder of the stem and gently scrape the gills away from the underbody of the mushroom cap. Discard gill scraps.

Chili-Rubbed Tilapia with Asparagus
We love tilapia in our house – it is so versatile and so yummy. Here it is spiced with chili powder and garlic, broiled and served atop steamed asparagus. Add some brown rice and you've got dinner!!

2 pounds asparagus, ends trimmed and cut into 2" pieces
2 tbsp chili powder
½ tsp garlic powder
¼ tsp salt
4 medium tilapia filets (~1 pound)

Preheat broiler to high. Combine chili powder, garlic powder and salt in a small bowl. Rub each filet with the spice mixture on both sides and place on a baking sheet sprayed with nonstick olive oil spray.

Broil on high until fish is cooked through, approximately 10 minutes. Steam asparagus until crisp tender (~ 6 minutes).

Serve 1 tilapia filet with ¼ of the asparagus.

Recipe makes 4 servings
211 Calories; 10 g Total Fat; 8 g Carbohydrate; 4 g Fiber; 26 g Protein

Broiled Honey-Soy Salmon
Delicious, delicate salmon marinated in a sweet, salty, tangy marinade. Easy enough for a quick weeknight dinner, but impressive enough for a dinner party! Leftover salmon is WONDERFUL in the Salmon Salad Sandwich recipe (see Lunch recipes), so make extra!

1 scallion, minced
2 Tbsp. reduced-sodium soy sauce
1 Tbsp. rice vinegar
1 Tbsp. honey
1 tsp. minced fresh ginger
1 lb. salmon cut into 4, 4-oz. portions
1 tsp. toasted sesame seeds (purchase pre-toasted seeds or see Helpful Hint below)

Whisk scallion, soy sauce, vinegar, honey and ginger in a small bowl until honey is completely dissolved. Place salmon filets in a 1-gallon size ziploc plastic bag. Add 3 Tbsp. of the sauce to the bag, seal the bag and toss to coat the fish with the sauce. Remove excess air from bag and allow fish to marinate in the bag inside the refrigerator for 15-30 minutes. Reserve the remaining sauce.

Preheat broiler to high. Line a small baking pan with foil and spray with nonstick cooking spray.

Transfer the salmon to the pan, skin side down. Discard the bag and the marinade. Broil salmon 4-6" from the heat source until cooked though (approximately 10 minutes). Remove skin from each salmon filet (it will pull away from the flesh easily. Drizzle with reserved sauce and garnish with sesame seeds.

Recipe makes 4 servings
223 Calories; 6.5 g Total Fat; 8 g Carbohydrate; 1 g Fiber; 25.5 g Protein

---

Helpful Hint: Toasting Sesame Seeds

Heat a small dry skillet over low heat. Add sesame seeds to the skillet and stir constantly until they are golden and fragrant, 2-8 minutes. Do not leave them alone – they can burn very quickly and then you have to start over.

Grilled Bruschetta Chicken
Angie found this recipe on Kraft Foods website, adapted it to fit the Release Plan and it became a quick family favorite!

1 lb. boneless skinless chicken breast cutlets
¼ cup light sun-dried tomato vinaigrette dressing, divided
1 tomato, finely chopped
½ cup part-skim mozzarella cheese, shredded
¼ cup chopped fresh basil
Preheat oven to 350°F.

Place chicken in a large resealable plastic bag. Add 2 Tbsp. of the dressing to the bag. Seal bag and toss to coat chicken evenly with dressing. Allow to marinate 30 minutes in the refrigerator. Remove chicken from bag. Discard bag and marinade.

Line a baking pan with foil and coat lightly with nonstick cooking spray. Bake chicken on baking sheet for 8 minutes.

Meanwhile, combine remaining dressing, tomatoes, cheese and basil.

Turn chicken over. Top with tomato mixture. Bake an additional 10 minutes or until chicken is cooked through.

Recipe makes 4 servings
240 Calories; 9.5 g Total Fat; 3 g Carbohydrate; <1 g Fiber; 34 g Protein

Tex-Mex Casserole
This is not really a "casserole," but it is a one pan meal and it makes enough for a small army and is quick and yummy!!

1-1/2 cups cooked brown rice
1-1/2 lb. lean ground beef
1 cup salsa
1 cup 2% cheddar cheese, shredded
1 15 oz. can black beans, drained and rinsed well
1 cup frozen green peas

Brown lean ground beef in a large skillet until no longer pink. Pour browned beef into a colander and rinse with hot water. Add back to the skillet and add rice, beans, salsa, cheese and peas. Heat over medium-low heat and serve when cheese is melted.

Recipe makes 6 servings
362 Calories; 16 g Total fat; 31 g Carbohydrate; 6 g Fiber; 25 g Protein

Sesame-Herb Crusted Mahi-Mahi
Delicious and elegant dish – another totally appropriate dinner party entrée.

2 Tbsp. lemon juice
2 Tbsp. extra-virgin olive oil
1 clove garlic, minced
Freshly ground black pepper, to taste
1 lb. mahi mahi, cut in 4, 4-oz. portions
2 Tbsp. toasted sesame seeds
2 tsp. dry thyme leaves
¼ tsp. kosher salt

Preheat oven to 450°F. Line a baking sheet with foil and spray lightly with nonstick cooking spray.

Mix lemon juice, oil, garlic and pepper in a small bowl. Place fish in a large, resealable plastic bag and add lemon juice mixture to bag. Seal and toss to evenly coat fish. Allow to marinate in refrigerator for 15-20 minutes.

Place toasted sesame seeds in a small bowl and mix with dried thyme leaves.

Remove the fish from the bag (discard bag and marinade). Sprinkle fist with salt and coat evenly with sesame seed/thyme mixture, covering the sides as well as the top.

Transfer fish to the prepared baking sheet and roast until just opaque in the center – 12-14 minutes.

Recipe makes 4 servings
270 Calories; 11.5 g Total Fat; 1 g Carbohydrate; <1 g Fiber; 37.5 g Protein

Deb's Delicious Chicken Enchiladas
This is comfort food at its best. Creamy, savory, spicy – absolutely delicious!!

2 lbs. boneless, skinless chicken breasts
2 cups reduced sodium chicken broth
½ small onion, chopped
8 oz. fat-free cream cheese, softened
1 tsp. ground cumin
1 10oz package frozen, chopped spinach (thawed and drained – see Helpful Hint on page 105)
8 large La Tortilla Factory whole wheat tortillas
1 10oz. can reduced fat cream of chicken soup
1 cup (8 oz) fat-free sour cream
1 cup skim milk
½ small jalapeno pepper, minced
½ cup 2% cheddar cheese, shredded

Preheat oven to 450°F.

Arrange chicken in single layer in a glass baking dish. Pour broth around chicken. Bake chicken until no longer pink in the center (internal temperature of 170°F), 30-35 minutes. Allow chicken to cool until you can handle it, then shred. Discard broth.

Reduce oven temperature to 350°F.

Mix shredded chicken, spinach, cumin, onion and cream cheese together. Divide this mixture into 8 roughly equal portions. Place one portion in each tortilla spread like a log across the diameter. Roll up and place in a 9" x 13" baking pan.

Whisk soup, sour cream, milk and jalapeno together until smooth and pour over tortillas. Cover baking pan with foil and bake for 40 minutes. Remove from oven, remove foil from pan and sprinkle with cheese. Bake uncovered for an additional 5-10 minutes until cheese is melted and lightly browned.

Recipe makes 8 servings
307 Calories; 10.5 g Total Fat; 30 g Carbohydrate; 12.5 g Fiber; 34 g Protein

Stuffed Peppers
These stuffed peppers are absolutely delicious – even our young son loves them – pepper and all!!

2 large bell peppers (any color)
½ cup onion, chopped
1 garlic clove, minced
1 cup cooked brown rice
2 cups tomato sauce, divided
½ cup reduced fat grated parmesan cheese, divided
1 large egg, lightly beaten
1 lb. lean ground turkey breast

Preheat oven to 400°F.

Cut bell peppers in half lengthwise. Discard seeds and membranes, leaving the stems intact. Place in a foil-lined baking pan sprayed lightly with nonstick cooking spray, cut sides up.

Heat large nonstick skillet over medium heat. Coat with cooking spray. Add onion and garlic to pan. Sauté for five minutes or until onion is lightly browned. Remove from heat and let cool.

Mix onion and garlic mixture with rice, 1 cup tomato sauce, ¼ cup parmesan cheese, egg and ground turkey in a large bowl until well combined. Divide the meat mixture into 4 equal portions.

Place 1 portion in each pepper half and press to fill entire pepper. Place each pepper half in the baking pan.

Pour remaining tomato sauce over peppers. Cover baking pan with foil and bake for 45 minutes. Remove foil cover from baking pan and sprinkle each pepper with remaining parmesan cheese. Bake for an additional 5 minutes or until cheese melts.

Recipe makes 4 servings
309 Calories; 5 g Total Fat; 29 g Carbohydrate; 4.5 g Fiber; 37 g Protein

Flank Steak Pinwheels
Delicious and easy, but an elegant enough presentation to serve at a nice dinner party!

2/3 cup sundried tomatoes (not packed in oil)
2 cups boiling water
1 lb. flank steak, trimmed of fat
1 clove garlic, minced
3 Tbsp. light herbed cheese spread (Boursin or Alouette)
1 cup baby spinach
½ tsp. kosher salt
½ tsp. freshly ground black pepper

Preheat grill to high.

Place sun-dried tomatoes in a bowl. Pour boiling water over them and allow them to sit until softened, about 10 minutes. Drain and chop.

Place flank steak between 2 sheets of plastic wrap. Pound each side of the steak thoroughly with the pointed side of a meat mallet until the steak is a uniform ¼" thickness.

Rub garlic over one side of the steak. Spread cheese in a 3" strip down the middle of the steak. Top cheese with sundried tomatoes and spinach.

Roll the steak tightly along a long edge, tucking in the filling as you roll.

Release

Carefully sprinkle salt and pepper on outside of the roll. Turn the roll so that overlapping edge is on top. Push 8 wooden skewers, evenly spaced, through the roll close to the overlapping edge to hold the roll together. Slice the roll into 8 equal portions, roughly 1 to 1-1/2" thick with a skewer in each. Lay slices on their side and push the skewer all the way though so there is skewer sticking out from both sides.

Oil the grill rack and grill 3-4 minutes per side for medium-rare. Turn with a spatula to avoid losing too much filling.

Remove skewers and let pinwheels rest for 5 minutes before serving.

Recipe makes 4 servings
328 Calories; 19 g Fat; 13 g Carbohydrate; <1 g Fiber; 25.5 g Protein

Deb Cheslow & Angie Flynn

Legal Disclaimer

All material provided within *Release – The Simple Success Solution for REAL and PERMANENT Weight Loss* is for informational and educational purposes only, and is not intended to provide the reader with medical advice.

This book is not a substitute for medical care nor is it a substitute for consultation with a healthcare professional. Please discuss all medical questions with your health care provider. Statements made in *Release – The Simple Success Solution for REAL and PERMANENT Weight Loss* are the opinions of the authors, based on research and personal experience because we have a long running passionate interest in health and wellness. However, we are not doctors.

The statements made within this workbook have not been evaluated by the Food and Drug Administration. These statements are not intended to diagnose, treat, cure or prevent any disease. YOU SHOULD ALWAYS SPEAK WITH A HEALTHCARE PROFESSIONAL BEFORE ALTERING ANY PRESCRIBED TREATMENT PROTOCOL.

This book was developed by Green Bubble Services, LLC d/b/a Deb Cheslow Consulting. The information provided herein is believed to be accurate at the time it was created and it was based on research and our best judgment. However, like any printed material, information may become outdated over time. Information within this book may contain technical inaccuracies or typographical errors, even though we have made our best efforts to avoid any such errors. If there is any doubt as to the accuracy of any claim or information in this book, the reader is responsible for verifying same against an alternative source.

All users agree that all use of this book is at their own risk. Deb Cheslow Consulting does not assume any liability for the information contained herein, be it direct, indirect, consequential, special, exemplary, or other damages; including intangible losses, resulting from the use or the inability to use our program.

Other Books by Deb Cheslow and Angie Flynn

The Simple Success Solution

The Simple Success Solution Companion Workbook

Overcome Dysthymia – Break Free and Create a Life You Love

www.myreleaseplan.com

release@myreleaseplan.com

(386) 308-1804

About the Authors

Deb Cheslow

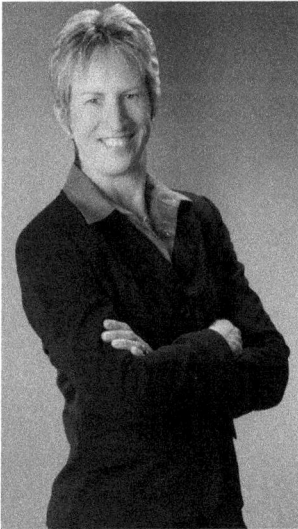

As an Air Force Instructor Pilot teaching airmen to fly advanced supersonic jets and a 3rd Degree Blackbelt in Karate, Deb Cheslow teaches how to reach goals that most people dream of yet few ever achieve - she gets RESULTS THAT COUNT!

Deb is not your typical motivational speaker; she over-delivers with motivation backed by sustainable results. Her entertaining and engaging style, packed with powerful ideas, leaves audiences not only motivated to reach their goals, but also equipped with the tools they need to get the job done. Deb teaches people how to bridge the gap between "information" and "action."

Best-selling author, speaker and corporate trainer, Deb Cheslow, considers it her mission to spread the message that a life of joy and abundance is attainable for anyone. Deb is known for her no-nonsense, direct approach. She believes audiences want, expect and deserve their speaker to be up front and honest about what works and what doesn't work. She guides companies worldwide in bridging the gap between the information they already possess and the actions they take on that knowledge (She calls it "The Information-Action Gap.").

Angie Flynn

Angie Flynn is the embodi-ment of the old adage "Life begins at 40." At age 45, Angie realized that she was a support-ing character in her life, not the star of the show.

There was no "intention" in her life, no direction – life was just happening around her and she was falling apart - mentally, financially, spiritually and phys-ically.

With a young son to care for, Angie Flynn knew something had to change – and in a BIG way. Enter Deb Cheslow, who introduced Angie to the concepts that they both now teach. In short order, Angie learned how to engage in the creative process to actively take control of her life. She learned how to break free from the limitations she placed on herself in her own mind, embrace the change that was necessary for her to Be, Do and Have what she really wanted in her life, and create a life that she LOVES. In a very short span of time, Angie was using this power to create an entirely new self-image and to overcome the life-long patterns that were keeping her from claiming her right-ful place, center stage, in a life of her choosing.

It is Angie's professional passion to share this information by creating tools to help others create the lives that, up till now, they may have only dared to dream about. As co-author of the best-selling book and the companion workbook, The Simple Success Solution; the book, Overcome Dysthymia - Break Free and Cre-ate the Life You Love, Angie shares her individual experiences and those of many clients by offering a dynamic, action-oriented process for taking you from where you are now to where you want to be.

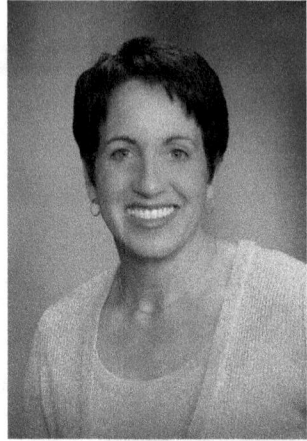

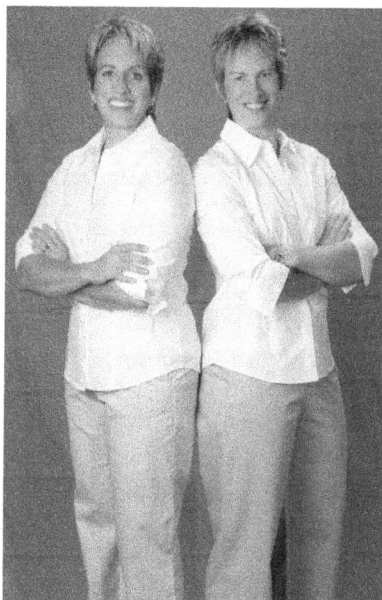

Deb Cheslow and Angie Flynn live in Ponce Inlet, Fla., with their family. They are authors of the bestselling book and the companion workbook, *The Simple Success Solution*; the book, *Overcome Dysthymia - Break Free and Create the Life You Love*; and their latest best-seller, *Release: The Simple Success Solution For Real and Permanent Weight Loss*. They share a passion for the martial arts, endurance cycling, health and wellness, and are avid weightlifters.

www.ingramcontent.com/pod-product-compliance
Lightning Source LLC
Chambersburg PA
CBHW051718020426
42333CB00014B/1050